Workbook for

PRACTICE & LEADERSHIP
IN NURSING HOMES

Building on Academic-Practice Partnerships

Andrea Yevchak Sillner, PhD, RN, GCNS-BC

JoAnne Reifsnyder, PhD, MSN, MBA, RN, FAAN

Ann Kolanowski, PhD, RN, FGSA, FAAN

Jacqueline Dunbar-Jacob, PhD, RN, FAAN

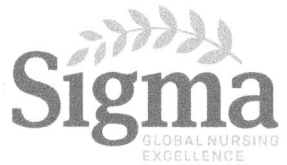

Copyright © 2026 by Sigma Theta Tau International Honor Society of Nursing

All rights reserved. This book is protected by copyright. No part of it may be reproduced, stored in a retrieval system, or transmitted in any form or by any means, electronic, mechanical, photocopying, recording, or otherwise, without written permission from the publisher. Any trademarks, service marks, design rights, or similar rights that are mentioned, used, or cited in this book are the property of their respective owners. Their use here does not imply that you may use them for a similar or any other purpose.

This book is not intended to be a substitute for the medical advice of a licensed medical professional. The author and publisher have made every effort to ensure the accuracy of the information contained within at the time of its publication and shall have no liability or responsibility to any person or entity regarding any loss or damage incurred, or alleged to have incurred, directly or indirectly, by the information contained in this book. The author and publisher make no warranties, express or implied, with respect to its content, and no warranties may be created or extended by sales representatives or written sales materials. The author and publisher have no responsibility for the consistency or accuracy of URLs and content of third-party websites referenced in this book.

Sigma Theta Tau International Honor Society of Nursing (Sigma) is a nonprofit organization whose mission is developing nurse leaders anywhere to improve healthcare everywhere. Founded in 1922, Sigma has more than 80,000 active members in over 100 countries and territories. Members include practicing nurses, instructors, researchers, policymakers, entrepreneurs, and others. Sigma's more than 600 chapters are located at more than 700 institutions of higher education throughout Armenia, Australia, Botswana, Brazil, Canada, Chile, Colombia, Croatia, England, Eswatini, Finland, Ghana, Hong Kong, Ireland, Israel, Italy, Jamaica, Japan, Jordan, Kenya, Lebanon, Malawi, Mexico, the Netherlands, Nigeria, Pakistan, Philippines, Portugal, Puerto Rico, Saudi Arabia, Scotland, Singapore, South Africa, South Korea, Spain, Sweden, Taiwan, Tanzania, Thailand, the United States, and Wales. Learn more at www.sigmanursing.org.

Sigma Theta Tau International
550 West North Street
Indianapolis, IN, USA 46202

To request a review copy for course adoption, order additional books, buy in bulk, or purchase for corporate use, contact Sigma Marketplace at 888.654.4968 (US/Canada toll-free), +1.317.687.2256 (International), or solutions@sigmamarketplace.org.

To request author information, or for speaker or other media requests, contact Sigma Marketing at 888.634.7575 (US/Canada toll-free) or +1.317.634.8171 (International).

ISBN: 9781646482313
PDF ISBN: 9781646482320

Publisher: Dustin Sullivan
Acquisitions Editor: Emily Hatch
Development Editor: Jillmarie Leeper Sycamore
Cover Designer: Kim Scott/Bumpy Design
Interior Design/Page Layout: Kim Scott/Bumpy Design

Managing Editor: Carla Hall
Publications Specialist: Todd Lothery
Project Editor: Jillmarie Leeper Sycamore
Copy Editor: Todd Lothery
Proofreader: Todd Lothery

DEDICATIONS

To improve the care and lives of people like my grandmother, who talked about her work as a nursing assistant giving her purpose and joy, and to later witnessing her living her last months with dementia in that same nursing home.
—Andrea Sillner

This book is dedicated to the diverse women and men who comprise the nursing home care force, providing expert care to our nation's most vulnerable citizens. And to the memory of my mother Anita, whose model as an endlessly compassionate and wise professional nurse inspired me to dedicate my life to caring for others.
—JoAnne Reifsnyder

To Cindy and David, and to the memory of Kollie and Mark, people whose lives give me purpose.
—Ann Kolanowski

To the memory of my husband, Rolf, who received care for his Parkinson's disease in nursing home skilled nursing services, thankful they are a valuable component of our healthcare system.
—Jacqeline Dunbar-Jacob

ACKNOWLEDGMENTS

Nurse educators play a crucial role in preparing learners for real-world healthcare challenges. Building academic-practice partnerships with nursing homes is a way for learners to develop hands-on skills in the care and management of some of the most complex persons: older adults. By immersing learners in the nursing home environment, we hope that learners can gain a deeper understanding of the complexities of nursing care in this setting, while ultimately improving outcomes for older patients.

This *Workbook* was created for nurse learners in academia and clinical practice by an interprofessional team of experts in the care of older adults. The precursor to this *Workbook* was the *Practice & Leadership in Nursing Homes: Building on Academic-Practice Partnerships* textbook, which came to fruition because of the Revisiting the Teaching Nursing Home Project and the original Teaching Nursing Project done in the 1980s. This body of work aimed to enhance nursing education by integrating nursing homes as active teaching environments, providing students with hands-on experience in nursing home settings to improve their clinical skills, aid in leadership development, and promote interdisciplinary collaboration while addressing the unique needs of older populations. Funded by the John A. Hartford Foundation, the Jewish Healthcare Foundation, The Henry L. Hillman Foundation, and the Independence Foundation, the initiative seeks to advance the quality of care for older adults through education and create sustainable partnerships between academic institutions and nursing home facilities. Through this project, the goal was to cultivate a new generation of nurse leaders prepared to meet the challenges of aging populations and complex care needs. This *Workbook* is another way to help meet these goals.

In addition, this *Workbook* is done in partnership with the Hartford Institute for Geriatric Nursing at the New York University Rory Meyers College of Nursing and the Jewish Healthcare Foundation. We would specifically like to thank Tara Cortes and Nancy Zionts for their energy, creativity, and dedication to this work and impacting the care and lives of older adults.

Finally, we would be remiss without acknowledging and thanking the many contributors to this *Workbook* who have rich, diverse experience in nursing home clinical care and nursing education, as well as operations, financing, policy, regulatory affairs, and technology in this setting. We give a special thank-you to our chapter leads Melissa Batchelor, Barbara Bowers, Julie Britton, Hillary Leger, Melissa McClean, Maureen Saxon-Gioia, and Nancy Zionts.

ABOUT THE EDITORS

Andrea Yevchak Sillner, PhD, RN, GCNS-BC, is an Assistant Teaching Professor at the Ross and Carol Nese College of Nursing at Penn State University. Her research and clinical focus are on improving communication between older adults, informal family caregivers, and formal healthcare providers. Her research has been supported by the Moore Foundation. Sillner also has a strong interest in preparing the next generation of nurses to be excited about caring for older adults and thinking about new ways to improve care through evidence-based practice and research in the undergraduate and graduate courses she teaches. Clinically, Sillner has had experience in acute and community-based settings of care and is board-certified as a gerontological clinical nurse specialist.

JoAnne Reifsnyder, PhD, MSN, MBA, RN, FAAN, is Professor, Health Services Leadership and Management, at the University of Maryland School of Nursing. She has held executive and leadership roles in hospice, hospice-related medication management, and skilled nursing. Her career clinical expertise is serious illness care for older adults. For 10 years, Reifsnyder served as the Chief Nursing Officer for Genesis HealthCare, the nation's largest skilled nursing provider. She is a Fellow in the American Academy of Nursing, was appointed by former HHS Secretary Alex Azar to CDC's Healthcare Infection Control Practices Advisory Committee to bring expertise in long-term care, is a member of NASEM's Roundtable on Quality Care for People with Serious Illness, and is an advisor to the John A. Hartford Foundation- and Jewish Healthcare Foundation-funded demonstration, Revisiting the Teaching Nursing Home.

Ann Kolanowski PhD, RN, FGSA, FAAN, is Academy Professor and Professor Emerita at the Penn State Ross and Carol Nese College of Nursing. She conducts research on nonpharmacological interventions for symptoms of distress and delirium in people living with dementia in nursing homes. Her research has been supported by grants from the National Institute of Nursing Research, the Alzheimer's Association, and the Hartford, Commonwealth, and Neuroscience Nursing Foundations. Kolanowski has published over 190 papers on dementia care in scientific journals and serves on many boards, including the Moving Forward Coalition, the Armed Services Retirement Home, and Kings College Board of Directors, as well as scientific advisory/consulting panels, including LINC-AD (Alzheimer's Association- and NIH-funded), EASE (Alzheimer's Association-funded), Impact of Nursing Home Leadership Care Environments and Health Information Technology on Outcomes of Residents with ADRD (NIH-funded), and the Teaching Nursing Home Project (Hartford- and Jewish Healthcare Foundations-funded). She was the recipient of the 2012 Doris Schwartz Gerontological Nursing Research Award and is a Fellow in the American Academy of Nursing and the Gerontological Society of America. Kolanowski was the founding Director of the Hartford Center of Geriatric Nursing Excellence at Penn State University.

Jacqueline Dunbar-Jacob, PhD, RN, FAAN, is Distinguished Service Professor and Dean Emeritus (Nursing) at the University of Pittsburgh. She was the founding Co-chair of the Implementation Steering Committee for the 2021 *Essentials* for the American Association of Colleges of Nursing. She was a participant in the NHLBI and NIA Working Conference on the Recognition and Management of Coronary Heart Disease and the Elderly (1985), National

Academy of Sciences Workshop on Adaptive Aging (2003), and NIH Office of Medical Applications of Research State of the Science Panel on Preventing Alzheimer's and Cognitive Decline (2010). Dunbar-Jacob chaired the Scientific Advisory Board for the NIH Roadmap Initiatives for the Patient Reported Outcomes Measurement Information System from 2004–2011. She was PI and CO-PI of the NSF project on the development of Personal Robotic Assistants for the Elderly (2000–2005). A registered nurse and licensed psychologist, she is a Fellow of the American Academy of Nursing, the American Psychological Association, the American Heart Association, the Society of Behavioral Medicine, and the Academy of Behavioral Medicine Research. She was principal for Revisiting the Teaching Nursing Home at the University of Pittsburgh (2021–2023) and consultant on the project to the Jewish Healthcare Foundation.

CONTRIBUTING AUTHORS

Melissa Batchelor (Chapter 12), PhD, RN-BC, FNP-BC, FGSA, FAAN, is an Associate Professor at George Washington (GW) University's School of Nursing and Director of GW's interdisciplinary Center for Aging, Health and Humanities.

Laura Block (Chapter 5), BS, BSN, RN, is a doctoral student at the University of Wisconsin-Madison School of Nursing and an RN with experience in post-acute and long-term care settings.

Marie Boltz (Chapter 4), PhD, GNP-BC, FGSA, FAAN, is a geriatric nurse practitioner with extensive, cross-setting clinical and administrative experience who has taught at all university levels (undergraduate, master's, DNP, PhD).

Barbara Bowers (Chapters 1 and 5), PhD, RN, FAAN, is Professor Emerita at the University of Wisconsin-Madison School of Nursing and Associate Editor of *The Gerontologist*.

Julie Britton (Chapter 10), DNP, MSN, RN-BC, GCNS-BC, FGNLA, is board certified as a clinical nurse specialist in gerontology and has spent the last 35 years working in post-acute and long-term care settings.

Sophie Campbell (Chapters 8 and 11), MSN, RN, CRRN, RAC-CT, CNDLTC, is Executive Director of the Pennsylvania Association of Directors of Nursing Administration (PADONA), through which Campbell supports nurse leaders and administrators in long-term care facilities in Pennsylvania. She is an approved provider of directed in-service education through the Department of Health and has worked as a licensed nurse in healthcare for more than 35 years, mainly in long-term care.

Joan Carpenter (Chapter 5), PhD, CRNP, ACHPN, FPCN, is an Assistant Professor at the University of Maryland School of Nursing, a health scientist at the US Department of Veterans Affairs, and a nurse practitioner with Coastal Hospice and Palliative Care.

Connie Cole (Chapter 5), PhD, DNP, RN-Gero, ANP-BC, ACHPN, is an Assistant Professor in the Division of Geriatric Medicine at the University of Colorado School of Medicine who has served as a nursing assistant, director of nursing, MDS coordinator, and nurse practitioner.

Kalei Crimi (Chapter 13), PhD, RN, is a postdoctoral scholar at the Center for Geriatric Nursing Excellence (CGNE) within the Ross and Carol Nese College of Nursing at Penn State University.

Emily Franke (Chapter 7), MSW, LSW, is a licensed social worker who currently serves as a Program Specialist supporting the Jewish Healthcare Foundation's Aging Team and the foundation's behavioral health initiatives.

Elizabeth Galik (Chapter 6), PhD, CRNP, FAAN, FAANP, is a Professor and Chair of the Department of Organizational Systems and Adult Health at the University of Maryland School of Nursing and a nurse practitioner who specializes in the medical and neuropsychiatric care of older adults with dementia.

Andrea Gilmore-Bykovskyi (Chapter 5), PhD, RN, is a practicing geriatric nurse and Associate Professor and Associate Vice Chair for Research in the BerbeeWalsh Department of Emergency Medicine at the University of Wisconsin School of Medicine and Public Health.

Hillary Leger (Chapter 3) is an undergraduate student at the NYU Rory Meyers College of Nursing, pursuing a degree in nursing and global public health.

Erin Kitt-Lewis (Chapter 2), PhD, RN, is an Associate Research Professor at the Penn State Ross and Carol Nese College of Nursing and the Associate Director of Education for the Tressa Nese and Helen Diskevich Center of Geriatric Nursing Excellence.

Caroline Madrigal (Chapter 4), PhD, RN, is a Nurse Scientist at VA Boston Healthcare System whose research focuses on the development and implementation of person-centered interventions, especially incorporating preference-based approaches as older adults navigate care transitions.

Kristin Mancini (Chapter 10), MSNEd, RN, CRRN, is Vice President, Staff Education and Policy Management, at Genesis HealthCare.

Melissa McClean (Chapter 6), MSN, CRNP, ANP-BC, CNE, ACHPN, is a board-certified nurse practitioner and nurse educator with advanced certification in hospice and palliative nursing who serves as a full-time faculty member at the University of Maryland, Baltimore School of Nursing.

Anne Bradley Mitchell (Chapter 9), PhD, CRNP, FGSA, is a nurse practitioner and undergraduate educator at the College of Nursing at Thomas Jefferson University and has been the Co-faculty Lead of the Jefferson Health Mentors Program for the past five years.

Christine Mueller (Chapter 7), PhD, RN, FGSA, FAAN, is a Professor at the University of Minnesota School of Nursing whose research career has focused on improving the care of elders living in nursing homes.

Wendy Ness (Chapter 10), MBA, NHA, QCP, has been with Genesis HealthCare for 15 years in many roles and currently serves as the Market President of Special Projects.

Michele Orzehoski (Chapter 9), DNP, MSN, RN, is a registered nurse with over 25 years of bedside experience and a full-time faculty member of the Thomas Jefferson University College of Nursing.

Anneliese Perry (Chapter 7), MS, NHA CECM, is the Program Manager, Aging Initiatives, at the Jewish Healthcare Foundation who has worked in both home and community-based services as well as long-term care.

Jennifer Pyne (Chapter 10), MSN, RN, is VP of Clinical Operations and Nursing Informatics at Genesis HealthCare.

Dr. Kiernan Riley (Chapter 13), PhD, BSN, RN, is an Assistant Professor at Fitchburg State University whose research has focused on improving the end-of-life period for vulnerable populations and community caregivers.

Maureen Saxon-Gioia (Chapter 7), MSHSA, BSN, RN, is a Nurse Project Manager for Aging Initiatives with the Jewish Healthcare Foundation.

Jennifer Sidelinker (Chapter 9), DPT, PT, is a Clinical Research Facilitator for Aegis Therapies with over 30 years of clinical and clinical leadership experience in a variety of older adult care settings.

Cathleen Soda (Chapter 10), RN, has worked at Genesis HealthCare for 26 years in multiple roles and currently serves as the Director of Patient Safety.

Brian Stever (Chapter 11), BSN, RN, RAC-CT, is the owner of Stever Advisors, LLC, where he consults on Medicare/Medicaid matters in long-term care.

Robyn Stone (Chapter 1), DrPH, is Senior Vice-President for Research at LeadingAge and Co-director of the LeadingAge LTSS Center at UMass Boston, a research center with offices in Washington, DC, and Boston, Massachusetts.

Julia Tague-LaCrone (Chapter 3), MPH, is a recent graduate of the NYU School of Global Public Health and a Graduate Research Assistant at the NYU Rory Meyers College of Nursing.

Jasmine Travers (Chapter 3), PhD, MHS, RN, AGPCNP-BC, is an Assistant Professor at NYU Rory Meyers College of Nursing and recently served on the National Academies of Sciences, Engineering, and Medicine Committee on the Quality of Care in Nursing Homes.

Nancy D. Zionts (Chapter 11), MBA, is COO/Chief Program Officer for the Jewish Healthcare Foundation and is responsible for the grant agenda for the foundation and its operating arms, Pittsburgh Regional Health Initiative and Health Careers Futures and WHAMglobal.

TABLE OF CONTENTS

About the Editors v
Contributing Authors vi
Introduction xiii

CHAPTER 1 **Nursing Essentials Checklist** 1
Brief Chapter Summary 1
Discussion Questions 1
NextGen NCLEX Style Questions 3
Case Study: Can Quality of Life and Quality of Care Coincide With Efficiency? ... 5
In-Class Activities or Assignments 7
Application of Content in the Clinical and/or Simulation Setting:
   Supporting Meaningful Lives in Nursing Homes 11

CHAPTER 2 **Creating a Culture of Care** 13
Brief Chapter Summary 13
Discussion Questions 13
NextGen NCLEX Style Questions 16
Case Study: Transforming Organizational Culture
   in Greenfield Nursing Home 17
In-Class Activities or Assignments 20
Application of Content in the Clinical and/or Simulation Setting:
   ANCC Pathway to Excellence Framework in Nursing Homes 22

CHAPTER 3 **Diversity, Equity, Inclusion: Staff and Residents** 25
Brief Chapter Summary 25
Discussion Questions 25
NextGen NCLEX Style Questions 27
Case Study: Implementing DEI in the Nursing Home Setting 28
In-Class Activities or Assignments 32
Role-Playing Exercise: Resident Refusal of Care Because of
   Race of Certified Nursing Assistant 32
Application of Content in the Clinical and/or Simulation Setting:
   Culturally Sensitive Considerations and Reflection in a Nursing Home ... 36

CHAPTER 4 **Person- and Family-Centered Care: Comprehensive Care Planning** ... 39
Brief Chapter Summary 39
Discussion Questions 39
NextGen NCLEX Style Questions 40

   Case Study: Upholding Resident Preferences in Skilled Nursing Care 42
   In-Class Activities or Assignments 44
   Application of Content in the Clinical and/or Simulation Setting:
    Person-Centered Care Reflection and Assessment in a Nursing Home 46

CHAPTER 5 Models of Nursing Care Delivery 52
   Brief Chapter Summary 52
   Discussion Questions 52
   NextGen NCLEX Style Questions 54
   Case Study: Team Nursing for Quality Care 56
   In-Class Activities or Assignments 58
   Application of Content in the Clinical and/or Simulation Setting:
    Hospice, Palliative, and End-of-Life Care 64

CHAPTER 6 Common Geriatric Syndromes 68
   Brief Chapter Summary 68
   Discussion Questions 68
   NextGen NCLEX Style Questions 70
   Case Study: A Nursing Home Resident Showing Symptoms of Frailty 71
   In-Class Activities or Assignments 77
   Application of Content in the Clinical and/or Simulation Setting:
    Reflecting on Geriatric Syndromes in Residents 79

CHAPTER 7 Developing the Workforce of the Future 78
   Brief Chapter Summary 78
   Discussion Questions 80
   NextGen NCLEX Style Questions 81
   Case Study: Stepping Into Leadership—Exploring the Role
    of a Director of Nursing in Long-Term Care 83
   In-Class Activities or Assignments 85

CHAPTER 8 Staff Development and Training 88
   Brief Chapter Summary 88
   Discussion Questions 88
   NextGen NCLEX Style Questions 91
   Case Study: Nurse Burnout in a Nursing Home Setting 92
   In-Class Activities or Assignments 96
   Application of Content in the Clinical and/or Simulation Setting:
    Nursing Home Staff Performance Evaluation 104
   References 106

CHAPTER 9 The Interprofessional Team and Collaborative Practice 107

Brief Chapter Summary 107
Discussion Question 107
NextGen NCLEX Style Questions 108
Case Study: Interprofessional Team Collaboration 109
In-Class Activities or Assignments 113
Application of Content in the Clinical and/or Simulation Setting:
 Goals of Care Conversation in the Nursing Home 120
Reference 119

CHAPTER 10 Regulatory Context 120

Brief Chapter Summary 120
Discussion Questions 120
NextGen NCLEX Style Questions 121
Case Study: Dining Observation in a Nursing Home 122
In-Class Activities or Assignments 124
In-Class Activities or Assignments for Learners Already Familiar
 With Nursing Home Setting 132
Application of Content in the Clinical and/or Simulation Setting:
 Five Scenarios for Identifying and Correcting Deficiencies in
 Care Provided in the Nursing Home 139
Reference 46

CHAPTER 11 Financing Senior Living Services and Long-Term Care 147

Brief Chapter Summary 147
Discussion Questions 148
NextGen NCLEX Style Questions 150
Case Study: The Benefits of Accurate Documentation in
 Skilled Nursing Facilities for the Minimum Data Set Process 151
In-Class Activities or Assignments 154
Application of Content in the Clinical and/or Simulation Setting:
 Balancing Clinical Care and Reimbursement Realities in a
 Skilled Nursing Facility 157

CHAPTER 12 Improving Quality in Nursing Homes 163

Brief Chapter Summary 163
Discussion Questions 164
NextGen NCLEX Style Questions 165
Case Study: Choosing a Quality Nursing Home for a Loved One
 With Dementia 166
In-Class Activities or Assignments 168
Application of Content in the Clinical and/or Simulation Setting:
 Using the NASEM Model of Quality in Nursing Homes to Design a
 QI Program to Reduce Resident Weight Loss 170

CHAPTER 13 Nursing Home Health Information Technology 173

Brief Chapter Summary 173
Discussion Questions 173
NextGen NCLEX Style Questions 177
Case Study: Coordinating a Specialist Appointment Using Health
    Information Technology in the Nursing Home 179
In-Class Activities or Assignments 183
Application of Content in the Clinical and/or Simulation Setting:
    Post-Clinical Reflection on Health Information Technology Usage 185
References 188

INTRODUCTION

Despite the growing demand for nurses trained to care for an aging population, the American Association of Colleges of Nursing (AACN) does not mandate geriatric-focused coursework or clinical experience for bachelor of science in nursing (BSN) programs (Mason et al., 2018). This gap in nursing education may lead to insufficient preparation of professional nurses in addressing the complex health needs of older adults, which is critical given the aging population in many countries (Stone et al., 2017).

In addition to a lack of formal geriatric curricula in many BSN programs, nurses in these settings often face complex clinical situations, including the management of geriatric syndromes, dementia care, and end-of-life issues, but are not always adequately prepared through formal training or ongoing professional development (Bowers et al., 2019; Stone, 2008). Comprehensive training programs focusing on geriatric care, including communication strategies and the management of chronic conditions, are essential to enhance care outcomes and improve the overall quality of life for older residents (Gaugler et al., 2020). This gap in specialized education can compromise the quality of care provided to nursing home residents, as nurses may lack the knowledge to effectively address the complex physical and mental health needs of the older adult (Liu et al., 2021). This impacts the quality of care provided to nursing home residents and contributes to high turnover rates, burnout, and lower job satisfaction among nursing home nursing staff (Bostick et al., 2006). Research indicates that many nursing homes cannot always support ongoing educational opportunities due to staffing and/or financial constraints, leading to insufficient support for nurses to stay current with evidence-based practices and advances in geriatric care (Harrington et al., 2012).

The Revisiting Teaching Nursing Home Project aims to address the critical gap in geriatric specialty education within nursing programs by fostering an academic-practice partnership between nursing schools and nursing homes. This initiative emphasizes the need for better-prepared nurses in nursing homes to manage the unique and complex care needs of older adults, including those with multiple chronic conditions, dementia, polypharmacy, and frailty (Gaugler et al., 2020). By integrating academic institutions with clinical practice settings, this project enhances nursing students' hands-on experience with elderly populations, providing them with the skills and knowledge to deliver high-quality care (Mason et al., 2018). Through this partnership, nursing schools can refine their curricula to include more geriatric-focused content, while nursing homes benefit from the partnership by getting students excited about working in this unique setting. In turn this can result in better-prepared professional nurses entering the nursing home to work, ultimately improving patient outcomes and nursing home staff outcomes, such as turnover (Stone et al., 2017).

The need to expose BSN nurses to issues faced in the nursing home and to improve professional training and development for those working in the setting led to the publication of *Practice & Leadership in Nursing Homes: Building on Academic-Practice Partnerships*. This innovative resource was designed to challenge nurse educators and learners to look beyond inaccurate negative connotations about nursing homes, to see how this growing healthcare arena can be ripe for nursing educational opportunities and rewarding careers for professional nurses. The textbook can be used in classroom and clinical courses as it provides foundational content on comprehensive care planning, models of care delivery, common geriatric syndromes, staff development and training, and nursing home financing, policy, and regulatory information.

The *Workbook for Practice & Leadership in Nursing Homes* is a supplement to the book and follows a similar format. It is meant to be a practical guide including reflective questions, case studies, pre/post-clinical content topics, classroom activities, and ways to apply content. Contributors to the *Workbook* represent dedicated educators, clinicians, and researchers focused on geriatrics.

WORKBOOK CONTENT

Professional organizations have identified basic competencies needed by professional nurses who practice in a variety of settings, including the nursing home. In 2021, the AACN released an updated version of *The Essentials: Core Competencies for Professional Nursing Education*, which reflects the evolving healthcare landscape and the need for nurses to be prepared for increasingly complex patient care. The revised framework outlines 10 essential domains that focus on advancing nursing education and practice to meet the demands of a diverse and aging population, as well as a rapidly changing healthcare environment. These domains include: (1) Knowledge for Nursing Practice, (2) Person-Centered Care, (3) Population Health, (4) Scholarship for the Advancement of Nursing Practice, (5) Evidence-Based Practice, (6) Quality and Safety, (7) Interprofessional Partnerships, (8) System-Based Practice, (9) Leadership, and (10) Professionalism. Each domain emphasizes a patient-centered approach that prepares nurses to lead across various settings, while focusing on improving health outcomes through collaboration, critical thinking, and continuous learning (AACN, 2021). These updates serve as a guide to ensure nursing education is aligned with the skills required for the future of healthcare delivery, with an emphasis on inclusivity, social determinants of health, and the integration of technology, all of which are relevant to those entering the field of geriatrics. Like the textbook, the *Workbook* emphasizes how the content and activities can help address these domains.

For the professional, practicing nurse continuing education (CE) ensures that RNs maintain current knowledge and skills. The American Nurses Association (ANA) emphasizes that CE helps nurses stay up to date with advancements in clinical care, technology, and evidence-based practices aligned with their specialty practice areas (ANA, 2021; Benner et al., 2010). The *Workbook* can help nurse learners in the professional setting align CE and/or professional development activities with learner needs about the complex nursing home setting and the residents within it.

Learners will explore the history of nursing homes and evolution into complex settings of care in Chapter 1 content and activities. Age-friendly care is the focus of Chapter 2, including What Matters, Medication, Mentation, and Mobility. Changes in the cultures, beliefs, and needs of persons cared for in the nursing home are explored in Chapter 3. Person- and-family centered care, with an emphasis on function-focused care, is the subject of Chapter 4. Various care-delivery models are covered in Chapter 5 activities. Chapter 6 focuses on the identification, assessment, and management of common geriatric syndromes. In Chapter 7, the learner is presented with the role of the advanced practice registered nurse in the nursing home. Nursing home staff development and performance is presented in Chapter 8 discussions and activities. The interprofessional team is an integral component of person-centered, nursing home care and is covered in Chapter 9. Quality and safety are covered in Chapter 10. Financial aspects of nursing homes are presented in Chapter 11 questions and learner activities. In Chapter 12, there is information on how to use knowledge gained through quality and safety measures to improve nursing home care. And finally, technology, clinical decision supports, and the electronic health record is explored in Chapter 13.

WORKBOOK ORGANIZATION

The *Workbook for Practice & Leadership in Nursing Homes* is organized with the following resources for each corresponding chapter of the *Practice & Leadership in Nursing Homes* textbook:

- Discussion questions
- NextGen NCLEX style questions
- Case study with application ideas
- Classroom activities
- Application of content in the clinical and/or simulation setting

Discussion Questions

Each chapter of the *Workbook for Practice & Leadership in Nursing Homes* contains at least one discussion question. The questions are designed to prompt discussion or reflection about chapter content. The discussion questions can be used in a variety of settings and ways to help learners reflect on the chapter content and emphasize student-driven learning.

NextGen NCLEX Style Questions

Each chapter of the *Workbook* contains NextGen NCLEX style questions. These questions can be used in a variety of settings and ways. For example, they can be incorporated into weekly quizzes or larger tests. They can also be used in synchronous and asynchronous class lectures or summaries as a self-check for learners.

Case Study With Application Ideas

The *Workbook* contains at least one case study with ideas for application for each chapter. A case study allows learners to use problem-based learning to promote thinking about real-world problems and solutions.

In-Class Activities

In-class activities are those tasks done by learners in an in-person or online class as part of applying practical components of the content included in the *Practice & Leadership in Nursing Homes* textbook. Each chapter of this *Workbook* includes several examples of classroom activities related to chapter content in the textbook.

Application of Content in the Clinical and/or Simulation Setting

The *Workbook* also includes ideas of how chapter content can be used in clinical and/or simulation settings. These applications are meant to be hands-on practical applications of textbook information focused on the nursing care of persons in the nursing home setting.

Our hope for the *Workbook for Practice & Leadership in Nursing Homes* is like that of the textbook: We want learners to be challenged when it comes to preconceived thoughts about professional nursing practice in the nursing home. Our hope is that through this *Workbook*, we can help learners in academia and professional settings do this more effectively and easily.

REFERENCES

American Association of Colleges of Nursing. (2021). *The Essentials: Core competencies for professional nursing education*. https://www.aacnnursing.org

American Nurses Association. (2021). *Nursing continuing professional development*. https://www.nursingworld.org

Bostick, J. E., Rantz, M. J., Flesner, M. K., & Riggs, C. J. (2006). Systematic review of studies of staffing and quality in nursing homes. *Journal of the American Medical Directors Association, 7*(6), 366–376. https://doi.org/10.1016/j.jamda.2006.03.013

Bowers, B. J., Esmond, S., & Jacobson, N. (2019). Nurse staffing in nursing homes: The role of training and staffing in improving care quality. *The Journal of Aging & Social Policy, 31*(1), 45–58. https://doi.org/10.1080/08959420.2019.1576719

Gaugler, J. E., & Kane, R. L. (2020). Improving care for elderly nursing home residents through geriatric training. *Journal of Aging & Social Policy, 32*(4), 300–315. https://doi.org/10.1080/08959420.2020.1740905

Harrington, C., Carrillo, H., & Wellin, V. (2012). Nursing home staffing, turnover, and case mix. *Journal of Aging & Social Policy, 24*(3), 192–203. https://doi.org/10.1080/08959420.2012.688173

Liu, W., Wang, C., & Chen, W. (2021). Barriers to and facilitators of geriatric care training in nursing homes: A systematic review. *Journal of Gerontological Nursing, 47*(5), 33–41. https://doi.org/10.3928/00989134-20210413-03

Mason, D. J., Leavitt, J. K., & Chaffee, M. W. (2018). *The future of nursing: Leading change, advancing health*. National Academies Press.

National Council of State Boards of Nursing. (2020). *Continuing education requirements for nursing licensure*. https://www.ncsbn.org

Stone, R. I. (2008). The nursing workforce in nursing homes: Can we meet the needs of an aging population? *The Journal of Aging & Social Policy, 20*(4), 248–268. https://doi.org/10.1080/08959420802356913

Stone, R. I., Reinhard, S. C., & Degenholtz, H. B. (2017). The nursing workforce and the challenges of caring for an aging population. *Journal of Aging & Social Policy, 29*(1), 59–73. https://doi.org/10.1080/08959420.2017.1364852

CHAPTER 1

NURSING ESSENTIALS CHECKLIST

–Barbara Bowers, PhD, RN, FAAN; Robyn Stone, DrPH

BRIEF CHAPTER SUMMARY

This chapter provides a historical overview of nursing homes in the United States, including how care provision has changed over time, the major legislation affecting care of older adults, and the growth and evolution of nursing homes. The chapter compares models of care and how each model affects resident quality of care and quality of life.

CHAPTER LEARNING OUTCOMES
- Trace the historical evolution of nursing homes
- Understand the "home" function of nursing homes and its relationship to quality of care and quality of life
- Describe models of care and the nursing home culture change movement

DISCUSSION QUESTIONS

Your instructor may use these questions as a group activity and class discussion, so consider the questions, record your responses below, and bring them to class.

1. What are some of the ways that nursing homes are unlike real homes?

   _____

   _____

   _____

   _____

2. How might these differences, related to a nursing home being unlike a real home, matter in terms of the residents' quality of life?

   _____

   _____

   _____

   _____

3. What can nursing homes do to increase the sense of home for nursing home residents?

4. What would be most important to your quality of life if you were in a nursing home?

5. What type of legislation do you think would help to improve quality of life for nursing home residents?

6. How does each model address quality of life? Do any address the issues that you would personally find the most important? If not, what would need to change?

NEXTGEN NCLEX STYLE QUESTIONS

1. What factor was primarily responsible for the shift from boarding homes that focused on social care for older adults to a medical model similar to hospitals?

    a. The distinction between deserving and undeserving poor

    b. The emergence of geriatric nursing as a specialty

    c. The rapid aging of the population

2. Which statement accurately describes the difference between for-profit and nonprofit nursing homes?

    a. Nonprofit homes generally have higher quality care and better clinical outcomes.

    b. Most nursing homes are nonprofit and affiliated with a religious organization.

    c. Nursing homes are increasingly shifting from for-profit to nonprofit status.

    d. Care quality in homes improves when they are purchased by for-profit organizations.

3. Which of the following statements about the GreenHouse care model is true?

    a. It is the most comprehensive culture change model.

    b. It includes consistent staff assignment to residents.

    c. It includes residents in decisions about their daily care.

    d. All of the above.

4. In the context of person-centered care (PCC), which statement is most accurate?

    a. It pays minimal attention to the medical issues of residents.

    b. It balances clinical/medical care with promoting resident quality of life.

    c. It has been standardized and can be easily integrated into daily care.

    d. Both b and c.

5. A nursing student is studying the history of federal nursing home regulations. Which of the following statements accurately reflects a key change in these regulations over time?

    a. Regulations have become less stringent, allowing for more flexibility in staffing.

    b. There has been an increased emphasis on resident rights and quality of care.

    c. Federal regulations no longer require documentation of resident care.

    d. Regulations have shifted focus from safety to financial management.

6. A nurse is educating a family about current filial obligation laws. Which statement should the nurse include in the teaching session?
    a. Filial obligation laws require children to provide all financial support for their parents.
    b. Filial obligation laws are federal mandates that apply universally across the United States.
    c. These laws vary by state and may affect financial responsibilities for nursing home care.
    d. Filial obligations only apply if the parent is living at home.

7. A nurse explains Medicare coverage to a patient being admitted to a skilled nursing facility. Which of the following aspects of coverage should the nurse emphasize?
    a. Medicare covers all long-term care needs without limits.
    b. Medicare will pay for nursing home care only if the patient has had a qualifying hospital stay.
    c. Medicare automatically provides coverage for all medications in nursing homes.
    d. Medicare does not require any documentation for reimbursement of skilled nursing care.

8. After learning about Hogeweyk Dementia Village in Amsterdam, a nurse reflects on its potential impact on dementia care. Which of the following features should the nurse identify as beneficial for residents with dementia?
    a. A simulated community environment that promotes independence
    b. Strict schedules and routine activities for all residents
    c. Isolated living arrangements to minimize confusion
    d. Limited staff interactions to encourage self-sufficiency

9. During a staff meeting, a nurse discusses the benefits of consistent assignment of direct care staff to residents. Which of the following benefits should the nurse highlight?
    a. Reduced staffing costs for the facility
    b. Decreased documentation requirements for care providers
    c. Increased familiarity and trust between staff and residents
    d. Greater autonomy for staff in decision-making processes

10. A nurse learns about a new nursing model that emphasizes continuity of information among care providers. Which of the following outcomes is most likely associated with this model?

    a. Improved overall care quality and resident satisfaction

    b. Fragmented communication leading to care errors

    c. Increased workload for nursing staff due to added documentation

    d. Decreased involvement of residents in their care decisions

11. A nursing team is implementing a relationship-centered team nursing approach. Which of the following practices should the team prioritize to improve care delivery?

    a. Focusing solely on task completion to ensure efficiency

    b. Assigning specific tasks without collaboration to enhance accountability

    c. Encouraging open communication among team members and residents

    d. Limiting staff interactions to maintain professional boundaries

CASE STUDY: Can Quality of Life and Quality of Care Coincide With Efficiency?

Narrative

You have recently taken a position in a local nursing home that has a reputation for providing high quality care. The nursing home has two sections: post-acute, a short-term section for people recovering from acute illnesses and planning to return home; and a long-term section for people who will not be going home. The nursing home is known for having very low hospitalization rates. That is, people in the post-acute section are rarely re-admitted to the hospital, and people in the long-term section are rarely sent to the hospital. As you know, this suggests that the care is probably very good. The staff at the nursing home are very proud of this.

You observe that the care is highly organized and that staff stick closely to their routine in order to be as efficient as possible. The shifts have even organized their care so that each shift tries to do what will make it easiest for the next shift to complete all their work.

Questions

Your instructor may use these questions as a group activity and class discussion, so consider the questions, record your responses below, and bring them to class.

For activities that will be done in class, as discussions or group activities, it is still beneficial to do some reflection before class to prepare.

1. You have learned about PCC and how important it is to residents. You are concerned that the staff are not sufficiently aware of this and may not have the flexibility in their care to provide PCC. How will you proceed?

   _____

   _____

   _____

   _____

2. How else might PCC be affected by the current care model?

   _____

   _____

   _____

   _____

3. How might you approach the staff to raise your questions? What do you think is the best way to engage them, generate some interest?

   _____

   _____

   _____

   _____

4. During a staff meeting you raise your concerns about residents' experiences and the importance of PCC. What are some ways that you might think about balancing a clinical care focus (which the staff are very proud of) with a more person-centered approach?

   _____

   _____

   _____

   _____

Resources

- Explore more about PCC as meaningful living here: https://pmc.ncbi.nlm.nih.gov/articles/PMC5102266/#:~:text=Person%2Dcentered%20care%20in%20nursing,her%20values%20and%20preferences%20first.

- A discussion of implementing person centered care: Rosemond, C. A., Hanson, L. C., Ennett, S. T., Schenck, A. P., & Weiner, B. J. (2012, July–September). Implementing person-centered care in nursing homes. *Health Care Management Review, 37*(3), 257–266. http://www.doi.org/10.1097/HMR.0b013e318235ed17.

- Some great culture change ideas: the National Long-Term Care Ombudsman Resource Center. https://ltcombudsman.org/issues/person-centered-care

IN-CLASS ACTIVITIES OR ASSIGNMENTS

Your instructor may assign these as in-class activities or as reflection activities done outside of class.

For activities that will be done in class, as discussions or group activities, it is still beneficial to do some reflection before class to prepare.

"What If" In-Class Activity or Assignment Questions: Emphasizing Person-Centered Care in Nursing Homes

In a nursing home setting, it is vital to prioritize PCC, which focuses on the individual needs, preferences, and values of residents. This approach not only enhances the quality of life for residents but also respects their autonomy and dignity.

The following "What if" scenarios encourage you to think critically about how to apply PCC principles in real-life situations and the necessity of balancing resident preferences with safety and health considerations.

Questions

1. What if a diabetic resident wanted a second piece of pie for dessert?

_____

_____

_____

_____

2. What if a resident's spouse (who pays the bills) wanted the resident to be out of bed by 7 a.m., but the resident wanted to sleep until 10 a.m.?

___

3. What if a resident wanted a beer but didn't have a medical order for one?

___

4. What if a resident did not want a male caregiver?

___

5. What if a resident wanted a bath five days a week?

___

Brain Drain Activity: Quality-of-Life Necessities

The purpose of this activity is to engage you in identifying and discussing quality-of-life necessities that contribute to the well-being of residents in nursing home settings. This will help you recognize both the essential elements of quality care and the current status of these elements in your environment.

Part 1: Individual Preparation

1. **Reflect:** Before the class begins, take a moment to reflect on what you believe are essential quality-of-life necessities for individuals, especially in a nursing home setting. Consider both physical and emotional aspects.

2. **List creation:** In the space below, write down five to seven quality-of-life necessities that come to mind.

    1. _____
    2. _____
    3. _____
    4. _____
    5. _____
    6. _____
    7. _____

Part 2: Group Discussion

Your instructor will guide a class discussion to share the quality-of-life necessities you identified in the first step of the activity.

During the discussion, document these responses, noting any patterns, common themes, or significant gaps in care that are identified during this discussion. You can use the space below for your notes.

Part 3: Focus on Nursing Home Settings

1. **Current environment analysis:** After the initial round of shout outs, shift the focus to the nursing home setting. Think specifically about the quality-of-life necessities that you observe in your current nursing home environment or from your experiences.

2. **Shout out again:** Repeat the shout-out process, this time focusing solely on the necessities that are present or absent in the nursing home. Consider discussion questions such as:

    a. What necessities are readily available to residents?

    b. Are there gaps in care that could be addressed?

    c. How do these necessities affect residents' overall well-being?

3. **Documentation:** Continue to document these responses, noting any patterns, common themes, or significant gaps in care that are identified during this discussion.

Part 4: Reflection and Debrief

Group reflection: After the shout-out sessions, the class will engage in a reflection discussion. Consider questions like:

1. Which necessities were most frequently mentioned?
2. What do you feel is lacking in the current nursing home setting?
3. How can we advocate for improvements in quality-of-life necessities for residents?

    You can use the space below for your notes.

Follow-Up Assignment (Optional)

After the class, your instructor may ask you to write a brief reflection (1-2 pages) on your insights from the activity. This could be done in class or as part of a take-home assignment or discussion forum. Your instructor may ask:

- Identify a quality-of-life necessity you believe is critical but often overlooked in nursing homes.
- Describe strategies you could implement in your practice to enhance residents' quality of life.
- Identify any specific changes you would advocate for based on your observations.

You can use the space below for your notes.

APPLICATION OF CONTENT IN THE CLINICAL AND/OR SIMULATION SETTING: Supporting Meaningful Lives in Nursing Homes

This assignment aims to deepen your understanding of what brings meaning to the lives of nursing home residents and how nursing staff can support these values in their daily care. You will engage directly with residents to identify their preferences and observe how these preferences are integrated into their care.

1. **Resident interaction:** Spend time with a resident and engage in a conversation about what brings them joy and meaning in their life. Consider questions such as:
    - What activities or experiences do you enjoy the most?
    - Are there specific people or memories that are especially meaningful to you?
    - How do you like to spend your day here?

2. **Staff awareness:** During your interaction, observe and ask about the staff's awareness of the resident's preferences. Identify:
    - Which nursing staff members (RNs, LPNs, CNAs) are aware of what is most important to the resident?
    - How do they integrate these preferences into daily care routines?

3. **Observational notes:** Take notes on how the staff interact with the resident and whether they incorporate what you learned about the resident's preferences into care practices. Pay attention to specific examples of how staff support residents' interests, such as:
    - Engaging in conversations about family or personal history
    - Facilitating participation in hobbies or group activities that align with the resident's interests
    - Providing personalized care routines that respect the resident's choices (e.g., preferred mealtimes, personal hygiene routines)

4. **Reflection questions:** After your interactions and observations, consider the following:
   - Is the resident's perspective and what is most important to them being addressed in their daily care?
   - Are staff members discussing how they incorporate resident preferences into care? If so, what do they say?
   - Notice any gaps—where could staff improve in recognizing and integrating these preferences into care?

5. **Post-conference discussion:** Prepare to discuss your findings in post-clinical conference. If resident preferences are not recognized or integrated into care, what do you think might be the reason? Consider factors such as:
   - Communication barriers among staff
   - Time constraints that limit individualized care
   - Lack of training or resources to support person-centered approaches
   - Organizational culture that may prioritize task completion over personalized care

6. **Identifying joy:** Can you identify at least three ways that nursing home residents find 'joy' in living? Consider the following prompts:
   - What specific activities, interactions, or moments did you observe that brought residents joy?
   - How did staff facilitate or enhance these moments of joy?

Provide specific examples from your clinical observations to support your answers.

This assignment emphasizes the importance of recognizing and integrating residents' preferences into their care. By understanding what brings joy and meaning to residents, nursing staff can create a more fulfilling environment that enhances the quality of life in nursing homes. Engage with residents meaningfully, reflect on your observations, and contribute to discussions that advocate for PCC practices.

CHAPTER 2

CREATING A CULTURE OF CARE

–Andrea Sillner, PhD, RN, GCNS-BC; Erin Kitt-Lewis, PhD, RN

BRIEF CHAPTER SUMMARY

Organizational culture (OC) refers to the shared values, beliefs, and behaviors that shape how members of an organization interact and work together. It influences everything from decision-making and communication styles to employee engagement and the overall workplace environment. OC in nursing homes often emphasizes person-centered care, fostering a supportive and respectful environment that prioritizes the dignity, preferences, and well-being of residents while encouraging collaboration among staff.

OC is important in nursing homes because it directly impacts the delivery of quality nursing care, resident quality of life, and the quality of the work environment for nursing home staff. Initiatives such as Age-Friendly Health Systems, Pennsylvania Revisiting the Teaching Nursing Home, and Pathways to Excellence are working to positively influence the OC of nursing homes.

CHAPTER LEARNING OUTCOMES
- Define organization culture
- Describe initiatives (Age-Friendly Health Systems, Revisiting the Teaching Nursing Home, Pathways to Excellence) that promote an OC of care
- Understand how a culture of care affects the delivery of quality care, resident quality of life, and quality of the work environment

DISCUSSION QUESTIONS

Your instructor may use these questions as a group activity and class discussion, so consider the questions, record your responses below, and bring them to class.

For activities that will be done in class, as discussions or group activities, it is still beneficial to do some reflection before class to prepare.

1. What does *organizational culture* mean to you, and how do you believe it impacts the quality of care provided in nursing homes?

2. How would you describe the OC in your clinical experience or current workplace?

3. What elements contribute to a positive OC in a healthcare setting?

4. Can you provide examples of how OC has influenced team dynamics or resident care in your experience?

5. Brainstorm three to five questions specifically geared for a future employer in the nursing home setting regarding their OC and how leadership and staff support it. Imagine that you were in a job interview and you wanted to know more about the OC where you are interviewing. Areas to consider for questions include:

    - The values and beliefs of the organization and how leadership demonstrates their commitment to them in the OC
    - How nursing staff are encouraged to contribute to the OC, especially in interactions with staff and residents and in person-centered care
    - How conflicts or challenges are handled, and the training available to nursing staff to ensure they fit within the OC and apply best practices in geriatric care

    Write your questions below.

    1. _____

    2. _____

    3. _____

    4. _____

    5. _____

NEXTGEN NCLEX STYLE QUESTIONS

1. The nursing team is discussing the possible effects of the low patient satisfaction rate. The staff started to list possible strategies to solve the problem(s) head-on. Should they decide to vote on the best change strategy, which of the following strategies is referred to this?

    a. Collaboration

    b. Majority rule

    c. Dominance

    d. Compromise

2. Nurse Miller is reporting off to Nurse Johnson at the nursing station, which is located in the middle of the unit. Nurse Patel, the RN supervisor, approaches the two nurses and interrupts the report to reprimand Nurse Miller about a medication error that occurred two days ago. What actions could Nurse Johnson do next?

    a. Ask the RN supervisor to meet with Nurse Miller in private after the report is over

    b. Walk away and let Nurse Miller be reprimanded in front of residents, family, and staff

    c. Suggest the nursing staff hold a meeting to discuss ways to create a just culture of care related to medication errors

    d. Verbally agree with the Nurse Supervisor as medication errors can have negative outcomes for residents

    e. Do nothing; you are not a supervisor and have little input in the culture of care

3. Overall, private reprimands are more likely to lead to positive outcomes, fostering better relationships and encouraging constructive feedback. The facility's leadership is reviewing the results of an anonymous survey about the OC at Celebration Estates Nursing Home. What is the first step the leadership could take to promote a just OC?

    a. Hold a staff meeting and share only the positive feedback

    b. Email the staff a summary of the results that includes the positive aspects and concerns of the organization

    c. Hold a staff meeting and question the staff about their concerns

    d. Make immediate changes to address the concerns

4. Nurse Habib is responsible for implementing a shared governance model at the Waterfront Nursing Home. Which of the following strategies should Nurse Habib use to help facilitate the implementation of the shared governance model?

    a. Hold a workshop to educate the staff about the shared government model

    b. Develop a mechanism for staff feedback

    c. Ask a close friend and coworker who works on the same unit to assist with the project

    d. Meet regularly with leadership and staff

5. Select all the characteristics of a just OC.

    a. Transparent

    b. Respectful

    c. Punitive

    d. Authoritarian

    e. Person-centered

    f. Inclusive

CASE STUDY: Transforming Organizational Culture in Greenfield Nursing Home

Introduction

Greenfield Nursing Home is not unlike many other nursing homes and has long struggled with a punitive OC, where mistakes are met with blame rather than opportunities for learning and improvement. This environment has led to high staff turnover, decreased morale, and compromised resident care. Recently, Greenfield Nursing Home has struggled with retaining and sustaining nursing staff, relying heavily on costly traveling staff.

In response, the administrative team at the nursing home has decided to make a shift towards a better OC, involving a sense of a just culture that emphasizes transparency, accountability, collaboration, and shared decision-making. To make this move, there will be a transition to a shared governance model involving all nursing and interdisciplinary staff.

Presentation of the Case

The nursing staff at Greenfield Nursing Home reported feeling undervalued and fearful of retribution for errors, which led to a culture of silence regarding mistakes. This punitive atmosphere resulted in a lack of open communication, affecting both staff satisfaction and resident care outcomes. It also resulted in a high rate of turnover of nursing staff. Upon reflection, the leadership team decided to adopt a shared governance model, aimed at empowering staff members to participate in decision-making processes and fostering a culture of transparency and accountability.

Key steps included:

- **Staff surveys**: Conducting anonymous surveys to assess staff perceptions of the existing culture and areas for improvement.
- **Focus groups**: Organizing focus groups to gather qualitative feedback from staff about their experiences and suggestions for creating a more supportive environment.
- **Pilot governance committees**: Establishing pilot shared governance committees comprising nursing and interdisciplinary staff to address specific issues such as staffing, safety protocols, and quality of care.

Action/Intervention

To implement the shared governance model, the following interventions were introduced:

1. **Education and training:** Workshops were held to educate staff about the principles of shared governance and just culture, emphasizing collaboration, transparency, and continuous improvement.
2. **Regular meetings:** Monthly meetings for the governance committees were established to discuss progress, share successes, and address challenges. Minutes from these meetings were shared with all staff to promote transparency.
3. **Feedback mechanisms:** A new anonymous feedback system was implemented, allowing staff to report concerns and offer suggestions without fear of retribution. This feedback was regularly reviewed by the governance committees.
4. **Recognition programs:** Initiatives were launched to recognize and reward staff contributions to quality improvement efforts, fostering a sense of pride and ownership in the care provided.
5. **Leadership support:** Leaders committed to modeling just culture principles by acknowledging their own mistakes and encouraging open discussions about errors as learning opportunities.

Conclusions

After six months of implementing the shared governance model, Greenfield Nursing Home began to see improvements in OC. Staff reported increased job satisfaction, higher engagement levels, and a greater sense of ownership over their work. The environment is starting to become more transparent and collaborative, leading to better communication and improved resident care outcomes. Although challenges remain, the transition toward a just culture is a promising step forward for the nursing home.

Questions

Your instructor may use these questions as a group activity and class discussion, so consider the questions, record your responses below, and bring them to class.

For activities that will be done in class, as discussions or group activities, it is still beneficial to do some reflection before class to prepare.

1. What are the key characteristics of a punitive culture, and how do they impact staff and resident care?

2. How can a shared governance model contribute to a shift from a punitive to a just culture in a nursing home setting?

3. What role does leadership play in fostering a just culture, and what strategies can leaders employ to support this transition?

4. How can staff feedback be effectively utilized to enhance the shared governance model and ensure ongoing improvements?

5. What are some potential challenges in implementing a shared governance model, and how might they be addressed?

_____

_____

_____

IN-CLASS ACTIVITIES OR ASSIGNMENTS

Group Activity: The 4Ms in the Nursing Home Brain Drain

Objective

By the end of this activity the learner will be able to apply the 4Ms in their practice. Learners will identify and list effective assessment strategies for the 4Ms—What Matters, Medication, Mentation, and Mobility—in nursing home residents.

Materials needed: Whiteboard or flip chart, markers, and handouts outlining the 4Ms. Alternatively, this may be done in an online shared document or a group discussion forum as part of a class.

Assignment Instructions

1. **Introduction:** Your instructor will begin with a brief review of the 4Ms framework as it relates to organizational care in the nursing home and how each concept is important in the health and well-being of nursing home residents. The 4Ms are: What Matters, Medication, Mentation, and Mobility.

2. **Group activity:** Students will be divided into small groups and each group assigned one of the 4Ms. Your group will be asked to brainstorm and list specific ways to assess their assigned 'M' in nursing home residents. Include outcome measures and reporting to quality control groups as part of the assessment. Your group should also think about both physical, hands-on assessments or tools and observational techniques.

3. **Sharing and discussion:** After the brainstorming session , the instructor may invite students to share their assessments within their groups and then write them on a whiteboard or flip chart. Alternatively, the instructor may ask each group to share their assessments with the class.

   Students will then be encouraged to discuss each group's findings.

4. **Application:** As a follow-up or additional assignment or activity, your instructor may provide you with a case study or resident profile of a hypothetical nursing home resident for assessment. You may be asked to apply the assessment strategies you just practiced in the group activity to evaluate the 4Ms for the resident. This may be an individual assignment or another group activity.

The following web-based resource may be useful for the 4 Ms activities/assignments presented above: https://www.ihi.org/sites/default/files/2023-09/AgeFriendly_4MsBySetting_FullGraphic.pdf

Role-Play Activity: Interaction Between a Registered Nurse, Licensed Practical Nurse, and Certified Nursing Assistant in a Just Culture Versus a Punitive Culture

Objectives
- By the end of this activity, nursing students will better understand the importance of OC in healthcare settings, as well as the need for effective communication and collaborative problem-solving in promoting a just culture.
- Nursing students will explore the differences between a just culture and a punitive culture through role-play, enhancing their understanding of communication, accountability, and teamwork in healthcare settings.

Roles: Registered nurse (RN), licensed practical nurse (LPN), and certified nursing assistant (CNA)

Activity Description
Your instructor will lead an in-class role-playing activity to understand the differences between "just culture" and "punitive culture" in a nursing home using a scenario involving a medication error or a patient care oversight.

Debriefing and Discussion
After all groups have presented, your instructor will lead a class discussion comparing the two cultures.

1. How did communication differ in the just culture scenario compared to the punitive culture scenario?
2. What impact did each culture have on team dynamics and patient safety?
3. How did the RN, LPN, and CNA feel during each scenario?

Optional Follow-Up Assignments
1. Creation of a teaching resource for residents, families, or clinicians in the nursing home such as a pamphlet, brief presentation, flyer, mini brochure, or a "tidbit" of information that staff can read on the go.
2. Journal reflection or discussion board post about what you learned regarding the impact of OC on nursing practice and patient care. Consider how you would approach similar situations in your future roles.

Resource

The Nursing Home Toolkit (found here: https://www.nursinghometoolkit.com/) can be used as a resource and for examples of content in this section or others.

APPLICATION OF CONTENT IN THE CLINICAL AND/OR SIMULATION SETTING: ANCC Pathway to Excellence Framework in Nursing Homes

By the end of this post-clinical conference discussion, you will identify elements that contribute to a positive practice environment and areas needing improvement.

Objectives

- Engage in a reflective discussion about clinical experiences in a nursing home, focusing on the ANCC Pathway to Excellence framework
- Critically analyze clinical experiences
- Understand the significance of the ANCC Pathway to Excellence framework
- Develop practical strategies to enhance the practice environment in nursing homes

Preparation

In class, your instructor will provide an overview of the ANCC Pathway to Excellence framework, highlighting its importance in promoting a positive practice environment in healthcare settings.

The framework includes the following key elements:

1. Shared decision-making
2. Leadership
3. Safety
4. Quality
5. Well-being
6. Professional development

Clinical Experience Reflection

After a recent clinical day in the nursing home, learners will participate in a class discussion. Areas of consideration will include shared governance, effective leadership, professional development opportunities, and recognition of staff efforts. Your instructor may use the questions below as a group activity or class discussion, so consider the questions, record your responses below, and bring them to class.

For activities that will be done in class, as discussions or group activities, it is still beneficial to do some reflection before class to prepare.

1. Which elements of the ANCC Pathway to Excellence framework did you observe during your clinical experience?

   _____

   _____

   _____

2. How did these elements contribute or how do you think they might contribute to a positive practice environment for both staff and residents?

   _____

   _____

   _____

3. Identify elements of the ANCC framework that you believe need improvement based on your experience and list these areas of improvement on the whiteboard, facilitating an open dialogue about their observations and insights. Consider the following:

   a. Were there any barriers to effective communication or collaboration among staff?

   b. Did you notice any gaps in leadership support or professional development opportunities?

   c. How could recognition of staff contributions be improved in the nursing home setting?

   _____

   _____

   _____

   _____

4. Brainstorm alternative strategies that nursing home staff (RNs, LPNs, and CNAs) could implement (action plan) to enhance their work environment based on the strengths and weaknesses identified. Areas to consider include:

    a. How can shared governance be strengthened among staff?

    b. What leadership initiatives could foster better communication and support?

    c. What recognition programs could be implemented to celebrate staff achievements?

    d. What is one way you can advocate for positive change?

    _____
    _____
    _____
    _____
    _____

Follow-Up Assignment (Optional)

Your instructor may ask you to develop your own action plan on how you can advocate for positive changes in your future nursing practice.

CHAPTER 3

DIVERSITY, EQUITY, INCLUSION: STAFF AND RESIDENTS

–Hillary Leger; Julia Tague-LaCrone, MPH; Jasmine Travers, PhD, MHS, RN, AGPCNP-BC, FAAN

BRIEF CHAPTER SUMMARY

This chapter defines and contextualizes diversity, equity, and inclusion (DEI) as it relates to the nursing home workforce. DEI is crucial to reduce inequities for both nursing home staff and residents. For example, certified nursing assistants (CNAs) are often underpaid, poorly treated, and subject to discrimination and racism by coworkers and residents. Nursing home residents who are Black and Latino are subjected to inequitable access to high-quality healthcare. All parties can benefit from increased knowledge of DEI, nursing students and nursing homes alike.

> **CHAPTER LEARNING OUTCOMES**
> - Define inequities, health disparities, and diversity, equity, and inclusion (DEI)
> - Understand staff and resident issues related to DEI
> - Propose ways to improve the nursing home environment so that it supports DEI

DISCUSSION QUESTIONS

Your instructor may use these questions as a group activity and class discussion, so consider the questions, record your responses below, and bring them to class.

For activities that will be done in class, as discussions or group activities, it is still beneficial to do some reflection before class to prepare.

1. What are some ways in which diversity can be increased in the nursing home workforce? (i.e., how do we encourage people from all backgrounds to apply and want to work in nursing homes?)

   _____

   _____

   _____

2. In the context of a history of mistrust between non-white patients and the medical field, how can nursing home staff build a relationship of trust with residents?

___

___

___

3. How do diversity, equity, inclusion, and belonging (DEIB) efforts influence policy development and financial reimbursement in nursing homes? Provide examples where possible.

___

___

___

___

4. Imagine a policy that ensures a resident's method of payment, whether private pay, Medicaid, Medicare, or other insurance, does not influence the quality of care they receive in a nursing home. How could such a policy promote equity in nursing homes and across the long-term care system?

Consider DEIB policy areas such as cultural competency, inclusive care planning, reporting discrimination, etc. And identify the key stakeholders within the nursing home and outside the nursing home that you would need to engage to make equitable care a reality.

___

___

___

___

NEXTGEN NCLEX STYLE QUESTIONS

1. A nurse is providing care in a nursing home with residents from diverse cultural backgrounds. Which of the following actions demonstrates the least DEI in the nursing home setting?

    a. Scheduling residents for the same activities to promote community building

    b. Listening to residents and relaying input forward to nursing care management

    c. Respecting the unique needs of each resident

    d. Encouraging residents to participate in a variety of activities

2. A nurse is assigned to care for a resident who only speaks Spanish. Which is the best practice for the nurse to use when communicating with the patient (Nursing Education Organization, n.d.)?

    a. Use the patient's English-speaking family as translators

    b. Speak slowly and loudly to the patient and avoid complicated words

    c. Use an interpreter service

    d. Postpone important conversations for their primary care physician to avoid miscommunication

    (Question adapted from https://nursingeducation.org/lms/Questions/topic/56)

3. How do diversity, equity, inclusion, and belonging (DEIB) efforts influence policy development and financial reimbursement in nursing homes? Provide examples where possible.

    _____

    _____

    _____

    _____

4. Imagine a policy that ensures a resident's method of payment, whether private pay, Medicaid, Medicare, or other insurance, does not influence the quality of care they receive in a nursing home. How could such a policy promote equity in nursing homes and across the long-term care system?

   Consider DEIB policy areas such as cultural competency, inclusive care planning, reporting discrimination, etc. And identify the key stakeholders within the nursing home and outside the nursing home that you would need to engage to make equitable care a reality.

   _____

   _____

   _____

   _____

5. A resident with a darker complexion has recently been prescribed new medication by their primary care provider and reports to the nurse that they are developing a rash. During the initial assessment the nurse did not see anything on the skin. Which of the following actions best demonstrates the nurse including DEI in the nursing home setting?

   a. Disregard the resident's statement

   b. Assess the rash then report to the primary care physician if there are concerns

   c. Tell the resident to give it time to resolve

   d. Report the newly developed rash to the primary care physician

6. During your daily rounds with the resident, the resident does not communicate any unusual preferences. The family of a Spanish-speaking resident expresses the concerns of the resident to you in English. As a nurse in a nursing home with a diverse population, describe the steps you would take to promote DEI among all residents.

   _____

   _____

   _____

7. A resident has requested to adjust medications or treatments according to cultural preferences. How can you, as their nurse, ensure their preferences are respected while promoting DEI?

_____

_____

_____

_____

CASE STUDY: Implementing DEI in the Nursing Home Setting

Introduction

ABC Nursing Home is a long-term care facility that serves a diverse population of residents. However, the workforce does not reflect the diversity of its residents, and the staff lacks the cultural competence necessary to provide equitable care to their entire resident population. As a result, ABC Nursing Home is struggling with issues related to staff turnover, low morale among staff, and poor quality of care delivery.

Presentation of the Case

This lack of DEI not only affects the staff but also has a significant impact on the residents of ABC Nursing Home. Residents with diverse backgrounds and cultural experiences may feel isolated or misunderstood by staff who do not share their backgrounds or understand their cultural practices. This can lead to a lack of trust in the staff and a feeling of neglect or discrimination. Furthermore, residents who do not receive equitable care may experience adverse health outcomes or a decreased quality of life.

Action/Intervention

To address these issues, ABC Nursing Home's leadership team decided to implement a DEI initiative aimed at increasing diversity, promoting equity, and enhancing inclusivity in the workforce. The initiative involved the following steps:

1. Assessing the current state: ABC Nursing Home's leadership team conducted an assessment using the Cultural Competence Assessment instrument to determine the current state of cultural competence and DEI in the workforce. The assessment revealed that ABC Nursing Home's workforce lacked diversity, and the staff did not have the cultural competence or sensitivity necessary to provide equitable care to all residents. The residents also reported feeling isolated or misunderstood by the staff.

2. Developing a DEI policy: ABC Nursing Home's leadership team developed a DEI policy that outlined the organization's commitment to increasing diversity, promoting equity, and enhancing inclusivity in the workforce. The policy included a plan to recruit and retain a diverse workforce, provide cultural competence training to staff, and ensure that all residents receive equitable care specific to their needs and preferences. The policy also emphasized the importance of creating a welcoming and inclusive environment for residents.

3. Implementing the DEI initiative: ABC Nursing Home's leadership team implemented the DEI initiative by recruiting a diverse workforce, providing cultural competence training to staff from experts in this area, and involving residents, families, and staff in care planning meetings. Recruitment efforts that ABC Nursing Home drew on included garnering referrals from staff already working at the nursing home, working with faith communities and people from diverse backgrounds who were connected to communities of diverse backgrounds, and providing benefits that appealed to people of diverse backgrounds such as childcare and transportation. ABC Nursing Home also provided resources and materials in languages that CNAs and other staff could understand and created opportunities for advancement and bidirectional communication. The initiative also focused on creating a welcoming and inclusive environment for residents, including celebrating cultural events and providing culturally appropriate care, food, and activities.

4. Measuring success: The ABC Nursing Home's leadership team measured the success of the DEI initiative by tracking metrics related to DEI in the workforce. The metrics included the diversity of the workforce, the percentage of staff who completed cultural competence training, resident satisfaction with the care they received, and staff job satisfaction and retention rates.

The DEI initiative at ABC Nursing Home resulted in several positive outcomes, including an increase in staff morale and job satisfaction, a decrease in turnover, and an improvement in the quality of care provided to residents.

Increase in staff morale and job satisfaction:

1. With a more diverse workforce, staff members are likely to feel more valued and appreciated, which can lead to higher morale and job satisfaction.

2. Providing cultural competence training can also help staff feel more competent and confident in their ability to provide equitable care to all residents.

3. How do diversity, equity, inclusion, and belonging (DEIB) efforts influence policy development and financial reimbursement in nursing homes? Provide examples where possible.

4. Imagine a policy that ensures a resident's method of payment, whether private pay, Medicaid, Medicare, or other insurance, does not influence the quality of care they receive in a nursing home. How could such a policy promote equity in nursing homes and across the long-term care system?

5. Consider DEIB policy areas such as cultural competency, inclusive care planning, reporting discrimination, etc. And identify the key stakeholders within the nursing home and outside the nursing home that you would need to engage to make equitable care a reality.

Decrease in turnover:

1. With higher staff morale and job satisfaction, turnover rates are likely to decrease. This means that ABC Nursing Home can retain experienced staff members, reducing the need to constantly train new employees.
2. Lower turnover rates can also lead to more consistent care for residents, as staff members have more experience and knowledge of each resident's unique needs.

Improvement in the quality of care provided to residents:

1. A more diverse workforce with cultural competence training can provide more equitable care to all residents, regardless of their background or identity.
2. Involving residents, families, and staff in care planning meetings can help ensure that each resident's unique needs and preferences are taken into account when developing care plans.
3. Providing resources and materials in languages that CNAs can understand can also help ensure that all residents receive clear and accurate information about their care.
4. The ABC Nursing Home's leadership team attributed these positive outcomes to the organization's commitment to increasing diversity, promoting equity, and enhancing inclusivity in the workforce.

Conclusions

The case study of ABC Nursing Home illustrates the importance of DEI in the nursing home workforce for both staff and residents. By implementing a DEI initiative, ABC Nursing Home was able to recruit and retain a diverse workforce, provide culturally competent care, and enhance inclusivity in the workplace.

Questions

Your instructor may use these questions as a group activity and class discussion, so consider the questions, record your responses below, and bring them to class.

For activities that will be done in class, as discussions or group activities, it is still beneficial to do some reflection before class to prepare.

1. Why was resident satisfaction an important measure to include when evaluating the DEI initiative ABC Nursing Home created?

   _____
   _____
   _____
   _____

2. How did collaboration contribute to the success of the DEI initiative?

   _____
   _____
   _____
   _____

3. How do we ensure the initiative remains successful long term?

   _____
   _____
   _____
   _____

IN-CLASS ACTIVITIES OR ASSIGNMENTS

ROLE-PLAYING EXERCISE: Resident Refusal of Care Because of Race of Certified Nursing Assistant

Objectives
- Identify real-life examples of discrimination in the workplace
- Understand strategies to respond to discrimination in the workplace

Example scenario: Resident is a non-Latina white individual who refuses services by a Latina CNA.

A Latina CNA enters the room of a non-Latina white older adult resident and greets her. The non-Latina white older adult does not greet her back instead asks why the CNA is in her room. The CNA introduces herself as "I am [insert name], and I am here to assist you with getting out of bed today and heading down to the breakfast room." The non-Latina white older adult says "Get out of my room" followed by a racial slur. The CNA respectfully exits the resident's room. The CNA explains the situation to the nurse managing the care of the non-Latina white older adult.

Background information: Approximately 60% of residents at ABC Nursing Home are Medicaid enrollees and the remainder are private pay. ABC Nursing Home is fully staffed with a diverse population of workers from different backgrounds.

Roles: Resident, certified nurse assistant (CNA), registered nurse (RN), nursing home manager/administrator

Activity Steps

Your instructor will lead an in-class role-playing activity to explore possible responses to the scenario.

- Read the case study thoroughly, including the background information.
- Discuss how each role could potentially react.
- Engage in a debrief of the scenario.

Discussion Questions

1. What should the nurse do in response to the situation?
    a. The nurse listens and tells the CNA she will deal with it later.
    b. The nurse listens and tells the CNA to switch the resident with a non-Latina white CNA.
    c. The nurse listens, notes the incident, and tells the CNA she will report it to the nursing home administrator. In the meantime, the CNA must return to the room and complete her task.
    d. The nurse listens, notes the incident, and tells the CNA she will report it to the nursing home administrator. In the meantime, a non-Latina white CNA will be sent into the resident's room.

2. The nurse reports the incident to the nursing home administrator. As a nursing home administrator, how can you intervene? Which options demonstrate best practices?
    a. **Option 1:** Set up a meeting with the CNA and tell her she will be permanently reassigned to other residents.

b. **Option 2:** Set up a meeting with the CNA and apologize for the situation. Consider hosting an orientation with DEI experts for residents and staff regarding reducing bias and improving DEI in the workplace.

c. **Option 3:** Include bias training for workers to be aware of best practices for these situations.

3. Debriefing and discussion:

    a. What were the most important parts of the case study?

    _____

    _____

    _____

    b. What were the conclusions drawn by this role-playing exercise? Consider resident-centered care.

    _____

    _____

    _____

    c. How can you, as a nurse or nurse administrator, demonstrate that you respect CNAs and residents?

    _____

    _____

    _____

Group Activity: Brainstorm Policies to Improve DEI in the Nursing Home Setting

The objective of this brainstorm activity is to engage learners in a rapid-fire brainstorming session where they can generate and share as many relevant concepts or terms as possible related to policies to improve DEI in a nursing home setting. This will encourage quick thinking, collaboration, and a deeper understanding of care practices.

Your instructor will lead the in-class brainstorming session and then lead a follow-up discussion on the results.

Brainstorm Questions

1. Come up with a mock policy for each of the following criteria:

    a. Consider a policy that increases the rate of reimbursement that nursing homes receive. What does this policy look like? What are the pros and cons?

    _____
    _____
    _____
    _____

    b. Describe a policy where a patient's payment method does not affect the quality of the care they receive. How would this increase equity across nursing homes?

    _____
    _____
    _____
    _____

2. For each of the policies mentioned in question #1, identify the target decision-makers you would want to engage to make this a reality. Consider lawmakers, insurance companies, advocacy groups, and other impacted groups

    _____
    _____
    _____
    _____

As a class, discuss the results of each group's brainstorming activity.

Summarize key concepts identified during the activity and consider how you might apply what you learned to your own practice.

APPLICATION OF CONTENT IN THE CLINICAL AND/OR SIMULATION SETTING: Culturally Sensitive Considerations and Reflection in a Nursing Home

This assignment could be used as a simulation scenario, an in-class activity, or in pre- or post-clinical conference. For practicing nurses, this could be used as a continuing education activity.

This activity will enhance nursing students' and practicing nurses' understanding and application of person-centered care catered to diverse backgrounds in a nursing home setting by supporting DEI.

Clinical Simulation Instructions

Activity Overview

1. Pre-assessment reflection
2. Resident assessment simulation
3. Group debriefing

Part 1: Pre-Assessment Reflection

Before conducting assessments with residents, nurses will engage in a reflective exercise based on two key questions. This will set the intention for their interactions. Each learner will take 5–10 minutes to answer the following questions in their journals.

Reflection questions:

1. How can I honor the preferences of residents and ensure their medical needs are met?

   _____

   _____

   _____

2. How will I accommodate residents' holiday observances? Consider varying holidays observed around diverse regions.

   _____

   _____

   _____

After individual reflections, students may be asked to share key points with a partner or small group to encourage dialogue about their thoughts and intentions.

Part 2: Resident Assessment Simulation

Nurses will participate in simulated assessments with actors or role-playing residents to practice their reflective insights.

Materials needed: Scenarios for role-playing (include a variety of resident backgrounds and needs)

Role-play scenario: A nurse informs a resident they will return in half an hour to collect blood work mandated by their physician. The resident has planned to attend an event in honor of Juneteenth/[insert any holiday] that was organized by the nursing home and will begin in 20 minutes.

Your instructor will lead an in-class role-playing activity to explore possible responses to the scenario.

Part 3: Group Debriefing

After the simulation, a debriefing session will allow learners to discuss their experiences, insights gained, and areas for improvement.

Materials needed: Whiteboard or flipchart, markers

Questions

Use the space below to record your notes from the debriefing session.

1. What strategies were effective in demonstrating DEI?

   _____

   _____

   _____

2. How did you incorporate the idea of accommodation into your interaction?

   _____

   _____

   _____

3. How might this activity change your approach in real assessments with residents?

___

___

___

By engaging in this reflective activity, nursing students, and practicing nurses will enhance their ability to provide person-centered care, ultimately improving the quality of life for nursing home residents. This practice will help you develop a deeper understanding of the importance of DEI in your daily interactions.

CHAPTER 4

PERSON- AND FAMILY-CENTERED CARE: COMPREHENSIVE CARE PLANNING

–Andrea Sillner, PhD, RN, GCNS-BC; Marie Boltz, PhD, GNP-BC, FGSA, FAAN; Caroline Madrigal, PhD, RN

BRIEF CHAPTER SUMMARY

Person- and family-centered care includes the principles of dignity and respect, information-sharing, participation, and collaboration. Person- and family-centered care are important concepts, even highlighted within the most recent American Association of Colleges of Nursing's *Essentials* (2021).

In the nursing home setting, person- and family-centered care can be operationalized through preference-based care i.e., the assessment and alignment of care with resident preferences for care and activities to cultivate a feeling of at-homeness and an individualized approach to care. Function-focused care is an important philosophy of care that offers practical approaches to help a person recover lost function and/or optimize their current function. Function-focused goals emphasize activities of daily living and engagement in what matters most to the individual, including meaningful activities and social engagement. Both preference-based care and function-focused care are aligned with the Age-friendly Health System 4Ms framework, through their consideration of what matters to the person and optimization of mentation (cognition and emotional well-being), mobility, and appropriate use of medication.

CHAPTER LEARNING OUTCOMES
- Define person- and family-centered care and the elements that comprise it
- Use tools to assess preferences for care and activities
- Adopt function-focused care as the foundation for nursing practice in nursing homes

DISCUSSION QUESTIONS

Your instructor may use these questions as a group activity and class discussion, so consider the questions, record your responses below, and bring them to class.

For activities that will be done in class, as discussions or group activities, it is still beneficial to do some reflection before class to prepare.

1. How can nurses partner with families to provide high-quality and person-centered care to nursing home residents?

_____

_____

_____

_____

2. What approaches can nurses use to support preference-based care for residents living with dementia in the nursing home setting?

_____

_____

_____

_____

By systematically integrating these strategies, nurses can create a supportive environment that honors the preferences of residents with dementia, ultimately enhancing their quality of life and well-being. Continuous evaluation ensures that care remains responsive to the evolving needs of the resident, making it a dynamic and individualized process.

NEXTGEN NCLEX STYLE QUESTIONS

1. A nurse is conducting an initial assessment of a new resident in a nursing home. Which action by the nurse best demonstrates person-centered care?

    a. Focusing solely on the resident's medical history

    b. Asking the resident about their daily routines and preferences

    c. Using a standardized assessment tool without personalizing it

    d. Relying on family members for all information about the resident

2. During a care conference, a nurse discusses a resident's recent decline in mobility. Which approach reflects a family-centered care approach?

    a. The nurse suggests that the family should look for a more active facility.

    b. The nurse invites the family to share their observations and concerns about the resident's mobility.

    c. The nurse informs the family of the medical interventions without seeking their input.

    d. The nurse decides on a new care plan without consulting the family.

3. A nursing student is observing an experienced nurse interact with a resident diagnosed with dementia. The experienced nurse uses reminiscence therapy as part of the assessment. What is the primary benefit of this approach?

    a. It allows for a comprehensive physical assessment.

    b. It helps the resident recall detailed medical history.

    c. It fosters emotional connections and improves communication.

    d. It ensures compliance with care protocols.

4. A nurse is developing a care plan for a resident who expresses feelings of loneliness. Which intervention best supports a person- and family-centered approach?

    a. Schedule daily group activities without considering the resident's preferences.

    b. Encourage family visits and help the resident maintain relationships outside the facility.

    c. Focus solely on medical interventions to address the resident's feelings.

    d. Limit interactions with other residents to minimize stress.

5. During a routine assessment, a nurse discovers that a resident's cultural beliefs influence their healthcare decisions. What is the most appropriate nursing action?

    a. Educate the resident about standard medical practices.

    b. Dismiss the resident's beliefs and proceed with the care plan.

    c. Collaborate with the resident and family to incorporate their cultural beliefs into the care plan.

    d. Refer the resident to a social worker for cultural concerns.

CASE STUDY: Upholding Resident Preferences in Skilled Nursing Care

Case Details

Resident name: Mrs. Rose McDonnell

Age: 78

Gender: Female

Background: Mrs. McDonnell had been residing in the independent living resident of a continuing care retirement community for the past three years. Known for her vibrant personality and active lifestyle, she often enjoyed participating in community events, gardening, and maintaining her social networks. Mrs. McDonnell was fully responsible for her ADLs and IADLs and prided herself on her regular and structured care routine.

Recent medical history: Following hospitalization for a severe bacterial infection, Mrs. McDonnell was transferred to the skilled nursing section for rehabilitation. Due to complications, she has been unable to return to her prior level of functioning and now requires 24-hour care and assistance with transfers. This sudden change has left Mrs. McDonnell feeling frustrated, isolated, and apprehensive about her future.

Questions

Your instructor may use these questions as a group activity and class discussion, so consider the questions, record your responses below, and bring them to class.

For activities that will be done in class, as discussions or group activities, it is still beneficial to do some reflection before class to prepare.

1. What are the primary preferences that Mrs. McDonnell expressed regarding her care and living situation?

   _____

   _____

   _____

2. What are the main challenges the nursing home must address to uphold Mrs. McDonnell's preferences?

   _____

   _____

   _____

3. What strategies can the interdisciplinary care team implement to create an individualized care plan that respects Mrs. McDonnell's preferences?

4. How can the nursing staff ensure effective communication with Mrs. McDonnell regarding her care and preferences?

5. What rehabilitation goals could be set to align with Mrs. McDonnell's desire for independence?

6. What steps can the care team take to advocate for Mrs. McDonnell's potential return to independent living?

By reflecting on this case study, learners will better understand the importance of person-centered care in skilled nursing settings. They will learn how to balance resident preferences with the realities of care policies and procedures, ultimately enhancing the quality of life for residents like Mrs. McDonnell.

IN-CLASS ACTIVITIES OR ASSIGNMENTS

Assignment: Create a SMART Goal and Care Plan for a Nursing Home Resident Using the 4Ms Framework

Students will develop a SMART goal and corresponding care plan interventions focused on one of the 4Ms of age-friendly health systems: What Matters, Medication, Mentation, or Mobility (see Figure 4.1). This exercise will enhance students' understanding of individualized care in a nursing home setting.

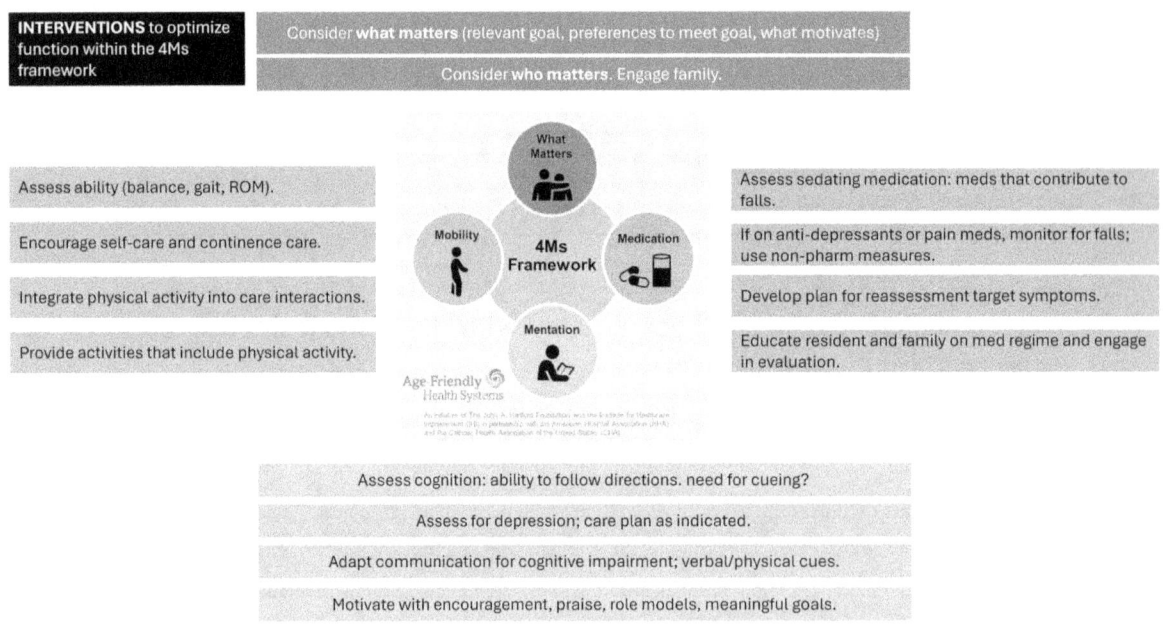

FIGURE 4.1 The 4Ms framework.

Assignment Instructions

1. Choose an area of focus: Select one of the 4Ms framework items to address for a hypothetical or real nursing home resident.

    - **What Matters:** Understanding the resident's goals, preferences, and values
    - **Medication:** Managing medications effectively and safely
    - **Mentation:** Assessing and supporting cognitive health
    - **Mobility:** Enhancing or maintaining physical mobility

2. Conduct background research: Review relevant literature and guidelines on best practices related to your chosen area of focus. Consider factors that may influence your chosen M for the resident population in a nursing home.

3. Develop a SMART goal: Create a SMART goal (Specific, Measurable, Achievable, Relevant, Time-bound) that addresses the selected M. Ensure the goal is patient-centered and aligns with the resident's preferences and needs.

   Example SMART goal format:
   - **Specific:** Clearly state what you want to accomplish.
   - **Measurable:** Include criteria to measure progress.
   - **Achievable:** Ensure the goal is attainable within the given time frame.
   - **Relevant:** Connect the goal to the resident's values and care needs.
   - **Time-bound:** Specify a timeframe for achieving the goal.

4. Create care plan interventions: Develop at least three specific interventions that support the achievement of your SMART goal. Each intervention should be:
   a. Evidence-based
   b. Patient-centered
   c. Feasible within the nursing home setting

   Example care plan intervention format:
   - Intervention: [Describe the intervention]
   - Rationale: [Provide evidence-based reasoning for the intervention]
   - Evaluation method: [Explain how you will assess the effectiveness of the intervention]

Assignment: Review and Revise Nursing Home Policy for Person- and Family-Centered Care

Learners will critically analyze a nursing home policy related to person- and family-centered care, identifying its strengths and limitations. They will then propose revisions or modifications to enhance the policy, ensuring it better meets the needs of residents and their families.

Assignment Instructions

1. Select a policy: Choose a nursing home policy related to person- and family-centered care. This could be a policy on resident assessments, family involvement in care planning, communication protocols, or any relevant area. Learners could also be given a standardized policy.

2. Review the policy: Read the selected policy thoroughly. Consider the following questions during your review:
   - What is the main goal of the policy?
   - How does the policy support person- and family-centered care?
   - Are there specific provisions for involving residents and families in care decisions?
   - Does the policy address the individual preferences and needs of residents?

3. Identify strengths and limitations: Create a list of strengths and limitations of the policy. Use the following format:
   - Strengths: (e.g., clear guidelines for family involvement, emphasis on resident dignity)
   - Limitations: (e.g., lack of flexibility in care plans, insufficient communication strategies)

4. Propose revisions or modifications: Based on your analysis, suggest specific revisions or modifications to the policy that could enhance person- and family-centered care. Consider how these changes could address the identified limitations. Ensure that your proposals are realistic and applicable within the nursing home setting.

5. Write a report: The report may be assigned as a written report, a discussion forum post, or a presentation as an in-class activity. Compile your findings into a report that includes the following sections:
   - Introduction: Briefly introduce the policy and its relevance to person- and family-centered care.
   - Policy analysis: Present your identified strengths and limitations.
   - Recommendations for revision: Detail your proposed changes and the rationale behind them.
   - Conclusion: Summarize the importance of enhancing person- and family-centered care in nursing home policies.

APPLICATION OF CONTENT IN THE CLINICAL AND/OR SIMULATION SETTING: Person-Centered Care Reflection and Assessment in a Nursing Home

This assignment can be used as a simulation scenario, an in-class activity, or in pre- or post-clinical conference. For practicing nurses, this could be used as a continuing education activity.

This simulation will enhance nursing students' and practicing nurses' understanding and application of person-centered care in a nursing home setting by fostering empathy, therapeutic partnership, and optimism.

Activity Overview

1. Pre-assessment reflection: Before conducting assessments with residents, nurses will engage in a reflective exercise based on three key questions. This will set the intention for their interactions.

2. Resident assessment simulation: Nurses will participate in simulated assessments with actors or role-playing residents to practice their reflective insights.

3. Group debriefing: After the simulation, a debriefing session will allow nurses to discuss their experiences, insights gained, and areas for improvement.

Part 1: Pre-Assessment Reflection

Before conducting assessments with residents, learners will engage in a reflective exercise based on three key questions. This will set the intention for their interactions. Each learner will take 5–10 minutes to answer the following questions in their journals or using another method like an online discussion forum:

1. How will I demonstrate empathy and respect for this person's uniqueness during the assessment process? Consider specific traits or life experiences of the resident.

   _____

   _____

   _____

   _____

2. How will I demonstrate that I value creating a therapeutic partnership with this person and their family? Reflect on how you can involve family members and respect the resident's input.

   _____

   _____

   _____

   _____

3. How will I demonstrate optimism for care and quality of living? Think about how you can encourage a positive outlook and highlight the resident's strengths.

___

___

___

___

After individual reflections, learners may be directed by their instructor to share key points with a partner or small group to encourage dialogue about their thoughts and intentions.

Part 2: Resident Assessment Simulation

Nurses will participate in instructor-led simulated assessments with actors or role-playing residents to practice their reflective insights.

Materials needed:

- Pre-printed or screen-sharing of scenarios for role-playing (include a variety of resident backgrounds and needs)
- Access to online tools:
    - Preference Based Living: https://www.preferencebasedliving.com/
    - Function Focused Care: https://functionfocusedcare.wordpress.com/
    - Institute for Patient- and Family-Centered Care: https://www.ipfcc.org/
    - Moving Forward Coalition Toolkit: https://movingforwardcoalition.org/
- Observation/reflection worksheet
- 4Ms framework handout (refer to Figure 4.1)

Role-Play Scenario

Your instructor will lead an in-class role-playing activity to explore possible responses to the scenario.

Name: Mrs. Lillian Martinez

Age: 87

Background: Retired teacher, bilingual (English/Spanish), and is widowed

Living situation: Recently admitted to the nursing home post-hospitalization for a mild stroke. She lives at home independently but has a daughter nearby that helps as needed. Her goal is to return home after her nursing home stay, but she is not certain that she will be able to do that.

Diagnosis: Hypertension, early-stage dementia, mild left-sided weakness

Likes/interests: Gardening, classical music, reading poetry, family visits (especially with her granddaughter), and she tends to speak Spanish when tired or emotional

Resident wishes: Lillian wishes to be outside without supervision at the nursing home to garden, but she is unstable due to the effects of the stroke. Wandering is also a concern considering the new environment of the nursing home and her dementia.

Concerns expressed by nursing home staff: Appears withdrawn, refuses morning physical therapy, has skipped a few meals, and becomes upset when routines change.

Scenario focus: Learners must assess Mrs. Martinez using a person-centered approach grounded in the 4Ms framework.

- **What Matters:** Understanding her goals, values, and what brings her joy or distress.
- **Medication:** Reviewing how her medications may impact her cognition or function.
- **Mentation:** Identifying early dementia symptoms and emotional wellbeing.
- **Mobility:** Encouraging functional movement while respecting her preferences

Simulation Instructions:

1. Your instructor will divide the class into small groups (3–4 people) and assign roles:
    a. **Resident (actor):** Learner portrays Mrs. Martinez, based on the scenario
    b. **Nurse (learner):** Conducts the assessment
    c. **Observers:** Provide feedback on communication and use of person-centered approaches

2. The Nurse learner conducts a live assessment of Resident, guided by:
    a. Pre-reflection insights
    b. The 4Ms (ask: *What matters most to you? What's hard about getting around? How are you feeling mentally and emotionally? How do you manage your care/medications at home?*)
    c. Tools from websites like the Preferences for Everyday Living Inventory (PELI) or Function Focused Care Coaching Tips

3. Observers complete feedback sheets:
    a. Did the nurse elicit "what matters most"?
    b. Were the residents' preferences respected, even if risky?
    c. Was the interaction empowering and empathetic?
    d. After the simulation, each group debriefs, discussing:
    e. What went well?
    f. What could be improved?
    g. How did the tools/resources support person-centered care?

Part 3: Group Debriefing

After the simulation, a debriefing session will allow learners to discuss their experiences, insights gained, and areas for improvement. Your instructor will lead the discussion with the following questions.

Materials needed: Whiteboard or flip chart and markers

Questions

Use the space below to record your notes from the debriefing.

1. What strategies were effective in demonstrating empathy and respect?

   _____

   _____

   _____

   _____

2. How did you incorporate the idea of partnership into your assessment?

   _____

   _____

   _____

   _____

3. In what ways did you foster hope and optimism during the interaction?

_____

_____

_____

_____

_____

4. Reflect on how this activity may have changed your approach in real assessments with residents.

_____

_____

_____

_____

By engaging in this reflective activity, nursing students and practicing nurses will enhance their ability to provide person-centered care, ultimately improving the quality of life for nursing home residents. This practice will help you develop a deeper understanding of the importance of empathy, partnership with nursing home residents and their families, and joy in your daily interactions.

CHAPTER 5

MODELS OF NURSING CARE DELIVERY

–Ann Kolanowski, PhD, RN, FGSA, FAAN; Barbara Bowers, PhD, RN, FAAN; Joan G. Carpenter, PhD, CRNP, ACHPN, FPCN; Connie Cole, PhD, DNP, RN-Gero, ANP-BC, ACHPN; Andrea Gilmore-Bykovskyi, PhD, RN; Laura Block, BS, BSN, RN

BRIEF CHAPTER SUMMARY

This chapter prepares nurses for care delivery in nursing homes by introducing them to models that guide practice in these settings. Because nurses may be less familiar with the unique goals and characteristics of the long-term healthcare system, they are contrasted to care delivery in acute care settings. Understanding the difference is essential for delivery of quality care and professional fulfillment. The importance of transformational leadership for achieving high quality long-term care and how that is enacted is discussed. Care-delivery models (CDMs) that are specific to long-term care and the role of the professional nurse in each are reviewed, including relationship-based team nursing, palliative and end-of-life, transitional, and dementia care delivery.

CHAPTER LEARNING OUTCOMES
- List CDMs common in nursing practice
- Describe the nursing role in palliative and end-of-life CDMs
- Outline the nursing role in transitional CDMs
- Summarize the nursing role in dementia CDMs

DISCUSSION QUESTIONS

Your instructor may use these questions as a group activity and class discussion, so consider the questions, record your responses below, and bring them to class.

For activities that will be done in class, as discussions or group activities, it is still beneficial to do some reflection before class to prepare.

1. How do the CDMs differ between nursing homes and hospital settings?

    _____

    _____

    _____

2. What is the primary goal of care in nursing homes compared to hospitals?

3. How does the primary role of the registered nurse (RN) differ in nursing homes and hospitals?

4. What competencies are needed for RNs working in nursing homes compared to those in hospitals?

5. How can you ensure that certified nursing assistants (CNAs) provide care that leads to the best clinical outcomes and quality of life for residents in long-term care settings?

NEXTGEN NCLEX STYLE QUESTIONS

1. The nurse manager in a nursing home setting is promoting high-quality, person-centered care. Which of the following activities would not be consistent with promoting this type of care?

    a. Knowing the unique capabilities of each staff member on the unit

    b. Seeking input on resident issues from all staff members

    c. Rotating staff assignments frequently to avoid burnout

    d. Acting as a mentor/coach to all staff

2. Which of the following best describes the team nursing approach?

    a. Relies heavily on a strong, decisive leader who makes decisions quickly and efficiently

    b. Is grounded in ongoing participation in decision-making from all staff

    c. Requires minimal skills or knowledge

    d. Is effective for managing clinical issues but is inconsistent with person-centered care

3. Which of the following communities is *least* likely to be considered underserved in terms of access to palliative care?

    a. Rural communities

    b. Nursing home residents

    c. Homeless populations

    d. Urban professionals

4. The nurse is discussing care options with the family of a resident diagnosed with terminal cancer. The family is considering whether hospice or palliative care would be more appropriate. Which of the following statements made by the nurse accurately describes the difference between hospice and palliative care?

    a. Hospice care is only for patients who are expected to live less than six months, whereas palliative care is appropriate for any stage of a serious illness, even if the patient is seeking curative treatment.

    b. Both hospice and palliative care focus on curing the illness, but hospice does not provide home care services.

    c. Palliative care is only offered in a hospital setting, while hospice care can be provided at home, in a nursing home, or in a hospice center.

    d. Hospice and palliative care are essentially the same, with the only difference being that hospice is covered by insurance and palliative care is not.

5. A nurse in a nursing home is approached by the family of a resident with advanced Parkinson's disease who is considering hospice versus palliative care. Which of the following is the most accurate explanation of the difference between hospice and palliative care?

   a. Hospice care is suitable when your relative decides to stop all aggressive medical treatment and is likely to live less than six months, whereas palliative care can be integrated at any time during the disease process, regardless of the expected outcome.

   b. Palliative care is typically short-term care that provides relief from acute symptoms, while hospice care is a longer-term solution that provides support until the end of life.

   c. Both hospice and palliative care are provided only in specialized facilities and focus primarily on pain management for terminally ill patients.

   d. You should consider hospice care when your relative is still undergoing treatments like chemotherapy or dialysis and switch to palliative care when treatments are no longer feasible.

6. Which of the following statements about palliative care is inaccurate?

   a. Palliative care team members address symptoms such as insomnia, anorexia, and delirium.

   b. Patients cannot receive palliative care if they are receiving curative treatments.

   c. Physicians, nurses, and physical therapists are often part of a palliative care team.

   d. Palliative care team members often provide emotional support.

7. The nurse is caring for a resident with advanced dementia who is experiencing a new behavioral symptom. The nurse knows that behavioral symptoms, or responsive behaviors, in dementia are most likely caused by which of the following factors?

   a. Unmet physical or psychological needs

   b. Personality and predisposition toward certain behaviors

   c. Underlying medical changes or needs

   d. Both a and c

8. The nurse is reviewing the medical chart of a new resident admitted to a nursing home following a lumbar compression fracture. Which of the following components of care is inconsistent with high-quality transitional care from hospital to nursing home?

   a. Structured hospital discharge summary

   b. Warm handoff from hospital staff

   c. Limited or no access to the hospital's electronic medical records

   d. Reconciliation of the resident's medication list

CASE STUDY: Team Nursing for Quality Care

Introduction

You have recently accepted a position at a nursing home as the unit manager for their dementia care unit. This is your first position in long-term care. You learn that the unit houses 30 residents with neurodegenerative diseases, mostly AD, in addition to other medical conditions and functional impairments. The Director of Nursing tells you that the staff on day shift (five CNAs and one LPN) need help dealing with resident agitation and aggression which has accelerated in the past few months around breakfast time and threatens staff retention because of the associated burnout.

In addition, the nursing home was cited for several deficiencies in their last survey related to 483.25 Requirement Quality of Care: Quality of care is a fundamental principle that applies to all treatment and care provided to facility residents. Based on the comprehensive assessment of a resident, the facility must ensure that residents receive treatment and care in accordance with professional standards of practice, the comprehensive person-centered care plan, and the residents' choices.

Action/Intervention

You realize that agitation/aggression are ways that residents with dementia communicate an unmet need. You also know that staff burnout can be associated with an inability to understand behavioral symptoms and effective ways to respond to these symptoms. Because you don't know the residents or the staff, you decide to take time to observe how care is typically delivered on this unit while getting to know residents and staff alike. Given that you are the new person on the block, you decide that the best way to do this is to help staff with delivery of direct care so you are seen as a team player, not a distant supervisor.

Over the next several days, you take time to help transport residents for their shower bath, help feed residents who need assistance, and make beds, all the while observing and communicating with residents and staff. Using the DICE approach (Describe, Investigate, Create, & Evaluate), by the second day you notice a pattern that seems to provoke symptoms in several residents. The five CNAs on this unit have organized their care so that all residents are out of bed and ready for breakfast by 7:30 a.m. They do this by working in teams of two, lifting residents OOB and whisking them into wheelchairs by 7 a.m. and having a third CNA circulate the unit while washing residents' face and hands and setting up the overbed table. Oral care is not done until later (if at all). Many of the residents are observed to be sleeping when their trays arrive at 8 a.m. and respond angrily when awakened for breakfast. Others attempt to remove the overbed table in order to ambulate freely on the unit, which is consistently discouraged before breakfast so that they "don't miss their mealtime." This, in turn, provokes angry outbursts that staff find difficult to handle.

How To Intervene

1. Continue to work as a team member with the staff and model alternate ways to respond to behaviors. Do this by example over time.

2. Call a huddle and introduce the DICE approach—help the staff see that their behavior of "needing to get work done"—may be precipitating the residents' behavior and making care more difficult to deliver.

3. Ask staff for volunteers who will work with you on a quality improvement project that has the dual purpose of reducing symptoms and improving the work environment.

4. Set up an all-staff education program on person-centered care using the preference-based living model to identify resident preferences for wake-up times and breakfast; consider a policy of consistent assignments, so staff get to know resident preferences; track symptoms and staff retention.

5. Discuss how new approaches can be integrated into care and ask for suggestions regarding the most effective ways to alter current routines.

Questions

Your instructor may use these questions as a group activity and class discussion, so consider the questions, record your responses below, and bring them to class.

For activities that will be done in class, as discussions or group activities, it is still beneficial to do some reflection before class to prepare.

1. What is important to consider when trying to change staff behavior?

2. How can you motivate staff to change behavior?

3. How will you approach staff so that they don't feel judged and criticized but are inspired and motivated to improve the way care is delivered?

4. What do you need to know about the staff in order to work with them effectively?

_____

_____

_____

5. How would you characterize the care that the current staff are using?

_____

_____

_____

6. How do you think a different model might address some of the current problems?

_____

_____

_____

IN-CLASS ACTIVITIES OR ASSIGNMENTS

Role-Playing Activity: POLST (Portable Orders for Life-Sustaining Treatment) Discussion in a Nursing Home Setting

This role-play activity helps learners understand the POLST process and practice communication skills in real-world situations they might encounter in a nursing home setting. The focus is on facilitating conversations about end-of-life care preferences between a resident, their family, and healthcare providers.

Scenario

In a nursing home, where the resident is seriously ill or approaching end-of-life care, the nurse meets with a family member and the resident to discuss and complete the POLST form.

Roles:

Resident: The nursing home resident has been informed about their terminal or serious condition and needs to make decisions about life-sustaining treatments. The resident's role is to communicate your preferences and ask questions about the POLST form.

Family member: The family member has strong emotional connections with the resident and might be concerned about the treatment options. The family member's role is to advocate for the resident's wishes, help them understand their options, and support their decisions.

Nurse: The nurse is responsible for explaining the POLST form and helping both the resident and the family member understand the medical options. The nurse needs to explain the choices clearly and supportively, ensuring that the resident's preferences are respected.

Materials needed: POLST form for your state. Access your state's POLST form at https://polst.org/state-polst-programs/.

Activity Description

Your instructor will lead an in-class role-playing activity to practice communicating with residents and family members about making end-of-life decisions and filling out the POLST form.

Debriefing Questions

After the role-play, the instructor will direct the group to come together for a debriefing session to reflect on the experience using the following questions. These might also be assigned as homework or a short reflective paper. Use the space below to record your notes from the debriefing session or reflection.

1. Resident's perspective: How did it feel to make decisions about life-sustaining treatments? Did you understand the options clearly? Were there any aspects of the form you found difficult to navigate?

   _____

   _____

   _____

   _____

2. Family member's perspective: How did it feel to advocate for the resident's wishes? Was it challenging to balance your feelings with the need to respect the resident's choices? How did you handle disagreements or uncertainties during the conversation?

   _____

   _____

   _____

   _____

3. Nurse's perspective: How did you feel explaining the POLST form? Were there any challenges in explaining complex options like CPR or feeding tubes? How did you ensure the resident and family felt comfortable with their decisions?

4. Discuss any challenges or emotional moments encountered during the role-play:

   a. Did the nurse encounter resistance from the family member about the resident's choices?

   b. Did the resident feel overwhelmed by the decisions they had to make? How did the nurse provide support?

   c. Did everyone feel heard and respected during the conversation?

5. Reflect on what went well during the role-play and what could be improved:

   a. Was the information about the POLST form clearly communicated?

   _____

   _____

   _____

   b. Were emotions appropriately addressed, especially when discussing end-of-life care?

   _____

   _____

   _____

   c. How could communication be improved in future similar situations?

   _____

   _____

   _____

Assignment: Create a Teaching Resource for Nursing Home Residents, Families, or Clinicians

The goal of this activity is for learners to develop an educational resource that can be used by nursing home residents, their families, or clinicians to improve understanding and communication about important topics in nursing home care, such as hospice and palliative care, advanced care planning, or managing chronic conditions. The resource should be easily accessible and practical, designed for quick reading or reference.

Assignment Instructions

1. Decide the audience: Decide who the primary audience for the teaching resource will be. Your resource can be designed for:

   ○ Residents: Older adults living in the nursing home who may need information on their care options, managing their conditions, or understanding their rights.

   ○ Families: Family members of residents who may have questions or concerns about their loved one's care and treatment choices.

- Clinicians: Nursing home staff, including nurses, CNAs, social workers, or other healthcare professionals who may need easy-to-digest, practical information to improve care delivery.

2. Identify the topic: Select a relevant topic based on the audience's needs. Some examples of topics include:
   - End-of-life care options: Explaining hospice and palliative care to residents and families.
   - Advance care planning: Educating families and clinicians on the importance of advance directives and POLST forms.
   - Chronic disease management: Tips for managing conditions like dementia, diabetes, or heart disease in a nursing home setting.
   - Pain management: How to recognize and address pain in elderly residents, especially those with cognitive impairments.
   - Resident rights: Key rights that nursing home residents should be aware of (e.g., autonomy, participation in care decisions, privacy).

3. You can use the Nursing Home Toolkit or the Hospice and Palliative Nurses Association's resources to find ideas and templates for your resource.

4. Choose format: Decide what format your teaching resource will take. Choose a format that fits the audience and the type of information you want to convey. Possible formats include:
   - Pamphlet: A printed, foldable sheet with concise information, suitable for quick reading
   - Flyer: A single page with key points, ideal for quick reference
   - Mini-brochure: A small booklet with detailed yet easy-to-read information that can be handed out to residents or families
   - Presentation: A short slide deck (e.g., for staff education or family meetings)
   - Quick "tidbit": A small, printed card or laminated sheet with one key piece of information or tip for staff to read on the go

5. Research the content: Gather relevant information from trusted sources to include in your resource. Focus on evidence-based, practical information that aligns with current best practices in nursing home care. Some key sources to consider include:
   - Nursing Home Toolkit: Offers practical strategies, tips, and resources for improving care in nursing homes (https://www.nursinghometoolkit.com/)
   - Hospice and Palliative Nurses Association: Provides guides and educational materials specifically geared toward nursing home care and palliative care (https://www.advancingexpertcare.org/education-events/nursing-resource-guides/)

- Centers for Medicare & Medicaid Services: For information on resident rights, quality of care standards, and regulations in nursing homes (www.cms.gov)

6. Create the resource: Using the information you have gathered, create the resource in the chosen format. Keep the following tips in mind:
    - Keep it concise: Ensure the resource is easy to understand and not overwhelming. Use bullet points, short sentences, and simple language.
    - Focus on key messages: Highlight the most important points about the topic. For example, if you're creating a pamphlet on palliative care, focus on what palliative care is, when it's appropriate, and how it can improve quality of life.
    - Make it visually appealing: Use colors, clear headings, and images (if appropriate) to make the resource visually engaging and easy to navigate. Keep the layout clean and well-organized.
    - Tailor it to the audience: For family members, consider including FAQs or concerns they may have. For staff, provide practical steps or action points. For residents, use reassuring language and explain the benefits of understanding their care options.
    - Provide contact information: If the resource is for residents or families, make sure it includes contact information for key staff members (e.g., care coordinator, social worker, or palliative care team) in case they have questions.

Examples of Potential Topics and Resources

- Pamphlet on palliative care options for residents and families
    - Overview of what palliative care is and how it differs from hospice care
    - When and why residents might consider palliative care
    - Practical benefits of palliative care (e.g., symptom management, emotional support)
    - Key contact information for palliative care teams

- Flyer on resident rights in the nursing home
    - Basic rights of nursing home residents (e.g., right to privacy, participation in care decisions, freedom from abuse)
    - Steps for residents and families to report grievances or concerns
    - Contact information for the ombudsman's office or resident advocacy groups

- Mini-brochure for clinicians on managing pain in dementia patients
    - How to assess and manage pain in patients with cognitive impairment
    - Common signs of pain in non-verbal residents
    - Medication and nonpharmacological interventions for pain management
    - Contact information for pain management specialists or palliative care team

- "Tidbit" card for nurses on POLST forms
    - Brief overview of what a POLST form is and why it's important
    - Key decisions that need to be made (e.g., CPR, feeding tubes, mechanical ventilation)
    - Steps to discuss the POLST form with residents and families
    - A quick checklist for nurses on ensuring the form is completed and stored properly

APPLICATION OF CONTENT IN THE CLINICAL AND/OR SIMULATION SETTING: Hospice, Palliative, and End-of-Life Care

Simulation & Assessment Activity

This scenario focuses on enhancing the nurse's skills in communicating sensitive information about health deterioration and the integration of palliative care into existing treatment plans, aiming to ensure a holistic approach that addresses both physical and emotional needs.

Role-Play Scenario

Your instructor will lead an in-class simulation activity to explore possible responses to the scenario.

Roles: Mr. Charles Williams (resident), family member of Mr. Williams, and nurse

Scenario

Mr. Charles Williams, an 82-year-old resident at your nursing home, has returned from the hospital where he was treated for pneumonia. He has advanced heart failure and mild cognitive impairment. Given the progression of his heart disease and the recurrent hospitalizations, it is crucial to discuss integrating palliative care into his current treatment plan to enhance his comfort and quality of life.

Debriefing Questions

After the simulation activity, the instructor will direct the group to come together for a debriefing session to reflect on the scenario using the following questions. These might also be assigned as homework or a short reflective paper. Use the space below to record your notes or responses.

1. How effectively do you think you communicated the necessity and benefits of palliative care to Mr. Williams and his family?

    _____

    _____

    _____

2. What were the challenges in discussing declining health and how did you address them?

3. How can you ensure ongoing comfort and dignity for Mr. Williams as his condition progresses?

Clinical Activity or Assignment: Dementia Care Interviews

Nursing students in clinical settings conduct family or friend caregiver interviews to ask about any behavioral symptoms they observed and ask them about their understanding of that symptom and what may have caused it.

Your instructor may assign this activity as a reflective journal entry or debriefing discussion with peers in class or in a discussion forum focused on the following prompts. Use the space below to record your responses.

1. Did the family/friend caregiver you met with recognize or identify behavioral symptoms?

2. What symptom did they identify and how did they describe this symptom?

3. What are ways their description/understanding of symptoms was similar to, or different from, information presented in Chapter 5?

Clinical Activity or Assignment: Transitional Care

Nursing students in clinical settings identify: 1) one recently admitted post-acute care resident and 2) one resident who was recently transferred from the nursing home to the emergency department or hospital.

The student will review the medical records for each resident with an eye for quality of communication, accuracy, and process improvement.

Your instructor may assign this transitional care activity as a written report, in-class discussion, or online discussion post. Use the space below to record your responses.

1. For the recently admitted resident, compare their 1) hospital discharge summary orders and medication list and 2) nursing home orders and medication lists. (Note: Some deviations may be purposeful and due to updates from nursing home providers). Key questions:

    a. Was the hospital discharge summary thorough and actionable?

    b. Has the nursing home completed quality checks of transfer of information into their medical record system?

c. Beyond orders and medications, what additional information is helpful/critical to caring for the resident, and how and where is this information transferred in your facility?

_____

_____

_____

2. For the resident transferred to the emergency department or hospital, review the nursing home medical record to determine reason for transfer, assessment and vitals leading up to transfer, and documentation using standardized tools. Key questions:

    a. Can you identify the reason for the transfer?

    _____

    _____

    _____

    b. Can you pinpoint any action that could have either prevented or aided the transition?

    _____

    _____

    _____

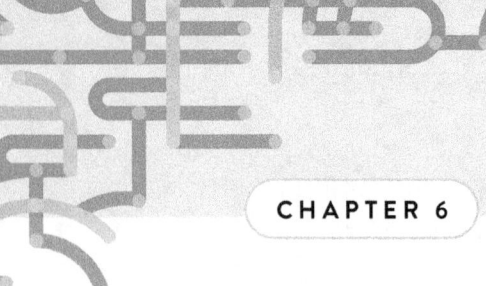

CHAPTER 6

COMMON GERIATRIC SYNDROMES

–Melissa McClean, MSN, CRNP, ANP-BC, CNE, ACHPN; Elizabeth Galik, PhD, CRNP, FAAN, FAANP; Andrea Sillner, PhD, RN, GCNS-BC

BRIEF CHAPTER SUMMARY

Unlike traditional chronic diseases, geriatric syndromes including cognitive impairment, malnutrition, frailty, falls, urinary incontinence, and nutritional deficits may create challenges for nurses practicing in nursing homes and long-term care settings. Thus, advanced practice clinicians, registered nurses, and nursing students in nursing homes should approach assessment, diagnosis, and management of these conditions with a more holistic and multifactorial approach. This chapter provides resources to increase understanding of common geriatric syndromes and enhance decision making with NCLEX style questions, discussion prompts, and a case study on frailty. It also includes learning activities for use in both classroom and clinical conference settings.

> **CHAPTER LEARNING OUTCOMES**
> - Describe geriatric syndromes common among older adults in nursing homes
> - Distinguish acute and chronic presentations of cognitive impairment
> - Appreciate that, although common, geriatric syndromes are not inevitable consequences of aging
> - Develop nursing care plans to prevent geriatric syndromes and restore optimal function and quality of life

DISCUSSION QUESTIONS

Your instructor may use these questions as a group activity and class discussion, so consider the questions, record your responses below, and bring them to class.

In the care of nursing home residents, it is important to differentiate between acute and chronic cognitive changes. Compare and contrast these two types of cognitive changes in older adults. Reflect on a scenario where a nursing home resident is presenting with signs of confusion. How would you assess whether the cognitive change is acute or chronic, and what immediate steps would you take to address the situation?

1. How might the clinical presentation of acute cognitive changes (e.g., delirium) differ from chronic cognitive changes (e.g., dementia, including Alzheimer's disease)? Write a comparison and contrast paragraph for your response.

2. What are the primary causes and risk factors for acute and chronic cognitive changes in nursing home residents? Write a paragraph for your response.

3. How would your approach to assessment, intervention, and care planning differ for a resident experiencing acute versus chronic cognitive changes? Write a comparison and contrast paragraph for your response.

4. Reflect on a scenario where a nursing home resident is presenting with signs of confusion. How would you assess whether the cognitive change is acute or chronic, and what immediate steps would you take to address the situation? Write a paragraph for your response.

___

NEXTGEN NCLEX STYLE QUESTIONS

1. An 82-year-old female resident in a long-term care facility has recently been admitted after a hip fracture. Over the past 24 hours, she has been increasingly confused, has difficulty focusing, and is unable to recognize her family members. Her vital signs are stable, and she does not have a fever. She has a history of hypertension and dementia. Which action should the nurse prioritize to manage this patient's symptoms?

    a. Administer a sedative to calm the patient

    b. Check for recent changes in medications that may contribute to delirium

    c. Encourage the family to provide familiar objects to the patient's room

    d. Begin a physical therapy plan to improve mobility and decrease confusion

2. A 74-year-old male resident of a nursing home has been diagnosed with functional incontinence, which is related to mobility issues and mild cognitive impairment. He is often unable to reach the bathroom in time due to difficulty walking and forgetting his need to void. Which of the following interventions is most appropriate to help manage this resident's incontinence?

    a. Insert a urinary catheter to prevent accidents

    b. Implement a scheduled toileting routine every two hours

    c. Encourage the resident to increase fluid intake throughout the day

    d. Limit fluid intake after 6 p.m. to reduce nighttime accidents

3. A 79-year-old female resident in a nursing home is at risk for falls due to muscle weakness and visual impairments. During morning rounds, the nurse observes that the resident frequently stands up without assistance and uses the bathroom without calling for help. Which intervention is the nurse's priority to reduce the risk of falls for this patient?

   a. Provide a bedside commode to prevent the need to walk to the bathroom

   b. Offer a walking cane to assist with mobility

   c. Encourage the resident to perform strength exercises to improve mobility

   d. Place the resident in a room closer to the nursing station to monitor her

4. A 76-year-old male nursing home resident with a history of frailty and chronic illness has been showing signs of unintentional weight loss, fatigue, and decreased appetite. He is able to eat but often forgets to eat or expresses no interest in food. Which intervention should the nurse implement to address this resident's nutritional deficits?

   a. Provide high-calorie, nutrient-dense snacks and meals throughout the day

   b. Increase fluid intake to promote hydration and prevent dehydration

   c. Offer nutritional supplements after each meal and snack

   d. Restrict the resident's meals to small portions to improve digestion

5. A 77-year-old resident in a long-term care facility has a history of Alzheimer's disease and hypertension. She has recently been prescribed a new antihypertensive medication. Her family reports that she has been more confused over the past two days, unable to recognize familiar people and agitated at night. Which nursing action should be taken first?

   a. Increase her dosage of antipsychotic medication to control agitation

   b. Review recent medication changes and assess for potential adverse effects

   c. Provide a quiet, dark room to minimize environmental stimulation

   d. Initiate a routine for family visits to maintain consistency and reduce confusion

CASE STUDY: A Nursing Home Resident Showing Symptoms of Frailty

Description

This case provides a comprehensive overview of a geriatric patient with multiple comorbidities and the complexity of managing her care in a nursing home setting. The nurse must assess and monitor all aspects of her physical, cognitive, and emotional well-being while involving the family in her care plan.

Name: Mrs. Anita Jackson

Age: 84 years old

Gender: Female

Admitting diagnosis:

- Atrial fibrillation (AFib)
- Hypertension
- Hypothyroidism
- Osteoarthritis of the knees
- Dementia (likely Alzheimer's disease)

Clinical Background

Mrs. Anita Jackson is an 84-year-old woman who was recently admitted to the nursing home following a brief hospitalization for dehydration and stabilization of her AFib. She had not been adhering to her prescribed medications, which led to her dehydration and exacerbated her AFib. Mrs. Jackson has a history of hypertension, hypothyroidism, osteoarthritis in her knees, and likely Alzheimer's disease.

Her primary informal caregiver is her niece, who is actively involved in her care and is concerned about her well-being, especially related to medication management and memory issues. Mrs. Jackson's cognitive decline has become more noticeable over the past several months, with increasing confusion, forgetfulness, and difficulty managing ADLs.

Current Medications

1. Amlodipine 5 mg daily
    - Indication: Hypertension
    - Class: Calcium channel blocker
    - Action: Lowers blood pressure by relaxing blood vessels, reducing the heart's workload

2. Warfarin (Coumadin) 2.5 mg daily
    - Indication: AFib for stroke prevention
    - Class: Anticoagulant
    - Action: Prevents blood clots from forming by inhibiting clotting factors

3. Levothyroxine (Synthroid) 75 mcg daily
    - Indication: Hypothyroidism
    - Class: Thyroid hormone replacement
    - Action: Replaces deficient thyroid hormone to normalize metabolism

4. Acetaminophen 500 mg every four to six hours as needed
   - Indication: Osteoarthritis pain in knees
   - Class: Analgesic
   - Action: Relieves mild to moderate pain and reduces fever

5. Donepezil (Aricept) 5 mg at bedtime
   - Indication: Alzheimer's disease (likely diagnosis)
   - Class: Cholinesterase inhibitor
   - Action: Increases levels of acetylcholine to help with cognition and memory in dementia

6. Furosemide (Lasix) 40 mg daily
   - Indication: Fluid management due to previous dehydration episode
   - Class: Diuretic
   - Action: Increases urine output to reduce fluid buildup and lower blood pressure

7. Omeprazole (Prilosec) 20 mg daily
   - Indication: GERD (gastroesophageal reflux disease), prevent ulcers
   - Class: Proton pump inhibitor
   - Action: Reduces stomach acid production to prevent irritation and ulcers

Physical Exam

General Appearance

Mrs. Jackson is an 84-year-old woman who appears slightly frail with a slow, cautious gait. She is alert but occasionally confused, especially when asked about the date or time. Her niece provides verbal cues to assist her with answers. Her hair is thin and slightly graying, and she wears glasses for reading.

- Vital signs:
  - Blood pressure: 148/90 mmHg (slightly elevated, considering her history of hypertension)
  - Heart rate: 88 bpm, irregularly irregular (consistent with atrial fibrillation)
  - Respiratory rate: 18 breaths per minute
  - Temperature: 98.7°F (37°C)
  - Oxygen saturation: 98% on room air

- Cardiovascular:
    - Heart: Irregularly irregular rhythm, no murmurs or gallops detected
    - Peripheral pulses: Weak, but palpable in all extremities
    - Edema: Mild bilateral edema in the lower extremities (may be related to her diuretic therapy or the effects of osteoarthritis on mobility)
- Respiratory:
    - Clear breath sounds bilaterally, no signs of respiratory distress or wheezing
    - No rales, rhonchi, or wheezing noted on auscultation
- Gastrointestinal:
    - Abdomen is soft, non-tender, and non-distended
    - Bowel sounds are present and normal
    - No signs of constipation, nausea, or vomiting
- Neurological:
    - Mrs. Jackson is alert but exhibits significant short-term memory loss, such as forgetting where she is and who is visiting her
    - She struggles to recall the names of familiar family members
    - Reflexes are intact but delayed
    - Strength is 4/5 in all extremities, with noted weakness in her lower extremities due to osteoarthritis
- Musculoskeletal:
    - Notable crepitus in both knees with limited range of motion
    - No significant joint deformities, though Mrs. Jackson complains of pain with movement
    - Difficulty with walking, especially when standing up or pivoting
- Skin:
    - Skin is slightly dry but intact without any signs of pressure ulcers or breakdown
    - No rashes or significant lesions

Assessment and Plan

- Cognitive decline: Mrs. Jackson's likely Alzheimer's disease is causing confusion and memory loss. This is managed with donepezil (Aricept), but the nurse and family must closely monitor her cognitive function. It's important to ensure she adheres to her medications, especially because she has had difficulty remembering them in the past.

- AFib: Mrs. Jackson is receiving warfarin for stroke prevention. Her anticoagulation therapy should be closely monitored, including regular INR checks, due to the potential for interactions with food and other medications (e.g., omeprazole may interfere with warfarin). Her AFib needs careful management to prevent complications such as stroke.

- Hypertension: Her blood pressure is somewhat elevated, likely due to the progression of her hypertension and possible nonadherence to her amlodipine regimen. This needs to be managed to prevent further cardiovascular complications.

- Osteoarthritis: Mrs. Jackson's knee pain and limited mobility require regular pain management (acetaminophen) and physical therapy. She should be assessed for assistive devices like a walker to help with mobility and reduce the risk of falls.

- Fluid and electrolyte balance: Furosemide was prescribed after her dehydration episode. The nurse should monitor her hydration status, electrolytes, and kidney function, as diuretics can increase the risk of electrolyte imbalances, especially in older adults.

- Medication adherence: Medication management is a priority, given Mrs. Jackson's cognitive decline and previous issues with not taking her medications as ordered. A medication reminder system or assistance from her niece may be beneficial in improving adherence.

Questions

Your instructor may use these questions as a group activity and class discussion, so consider the questions, record your responses below, and bring them to class.

For activities that will be done in class, as discussions or group activities, it is still beneficial to do some reflection before class to prepare.

1. What is the primary nursing assessment tool used in nursing homes to assess fall risk in older adults, and why is it important for Mrs. Jackson's care?

2. Based on Mrs. Jackson's condition, what specific factors should be considered when assessing her risk for falls?

3. What specific interventions should be implemented based on the fall risk assessment for Mrs. Jackson?

4. What role does Mrs. Jackson's niece play in the fall prevention strategy, and how can the nurse support her?

5. Mrs. Jackson is taking furosemide (Lasix), which can cause dizziness and increase her risk of falls. What nursing actions can help minimize the fall risk associated with this medication?

6. How would you assess the effectiveness of the fall prevention interventions in Mrs. Jackson's care plan?

IN-CLASS ACTIVITIES OR ASSIGNMENTS

Your instructor may assign these as in-class activities or as reflection activities done outside of class.

For activities that will be done in class, as discussions or group activities, it is still beneficial to do some reflection before class to prepare.

Role-Play Activity: Geriatric Syndrome Assessment and Care Planning

The goal of this role-play activity is to help nursing students practice assessing common geriatric syndromes (cognitive impairment, nutritional deficits, frailty, and sarcopenia) and develop nursing diagnoses, interventions, and goals based on their findings. Students will learn how to collaborate and create a care plan that addresses the unique needs of older adults with these syndromes.

Objectives

- Assessment skills: Students will practice performing comprehensive assessments for common geriatric syndromes and learn how to apply appropriate questions and observation techniques.
- Critical thinking: Students will enhance their ability to develop personalized care plans by identifying key nursing diagnoses, interventions, and goals for older adults with complex needs.
- Collaborative care planning: Students will work together to develop holistic, patient-centered care plans, reinforcing the importance of teamwork in nursing practice.

Scenario: A nurse uses a standardized assessment tool or asks a series of questions to evaluate a specific geriatric syndrome (cognitive impairment, nutritional deficits, frailty, sarcopenia) in a patient.

Roles: Nurse, patient

Activity Steps

1. Your instructor will lead an in-class role-playing activity to explore possible responses to the scenario.
2. After the role-play, the paired learners will create a care plan including the following:
    a. Nursing diagnoses: Based on the findings of each assessment, learners should formulate at least two nursing diagnoses for each geriatric syndrome (one for each student's role-played syndrome).
    b. Nursing interventions: For each diagnosis, identify at least two nursing interventions.
    c. Goals: For each intervention, identify both a short-term and a long-term goal.
3. Once pairs have completed their care plans, the class will come together and share their nursing diagnoses, interventions, and goals with the larger group.

Debriefing

After the role-play, the instructor will direct the group to come together for a debriefing session to reflect on the experience using the following questions. These might also be assigned as homework or a short reflective paper. Use the space below to record your notes from the debriefing session or reflection.

1. What did you learn about the challenges of assessing geriatric syndromes in real-life scenarios?

2. How did the role-play help you better understand the complexities of managing multiple geriatric syndromes?

3. Which nursing interventions do you feel most confident in implementing based on your learning today?

APPLICATION OF CONTENT IN THE CLINICAL AND/OR SIMULATION SETTING: Reflecting on Geriatric Syndromes in Residents

Post-Clinical Conference Activity

The purpose of this post-clinical conference activity is to provide nursing students an opportunity to reflect upon their clinical experience with elderly residents, specifically those exhibiting at least one geriatric syndrome. Through a group discussion, students will analyze current care strategies, share insights, and collaboratively propose additional nursing assessments or interventions.

Objectives

- Clinical reasoning: Apply clinical reasoning to assess the care needs of residents with geriatric syndromes and evaluate whether current nursing interventions are adequate.

- Collaboration and advocacy: Practice collaborating with the healthcare team, including other disciplines, to enhance care for older adults.

- Reflective practice: Reflect on their experiences to identify areas for growth in their ability to assess and manage geriatric syndromes in long-term care settings.

Activity Instructions

1. Learner reflection:

   Choose one resident you cared for during the clinical day who presented with at least one geriatric syndrome (e.g., delirium, incontinence, frailty, falls, nutritional deficits, or cognitive impairment).

   Reflect on the following aspects:

   a. What geriatric syndrome(s) did the resident exhibit?

   b. What assessments were conducted or interventions already in place for this syndrome?

   c. Were there any challenges encountered when providing care for this syndrome?

   d. How did the resident's condition impact their quality of life, and how was this communicated to the healthcare team?

2. Prepare to share:

   Jot down notes about the care you provided and your observations. Focus on the nursing interventions you implemented (e.g., pain management, mobility assistance, medication adjustments) and any nursing assessments that were completed during the shift (e.g., fall risk assessment, nutritional screening, cognitive assessment). You can use the space below to make your notes.

   _____

   _____

   _____

   _____

3. Group discussion:

   In the clinical group, each learner will briefly present their chosen resident's condition, discussing the geriatric syndrome, the nursing interventions provided, and the current care plan in place.

   After each presentation, the group will engage in a guided discussion.

Group Discussion Questions

Your instructor may use these questions as a group activity and class discussion, so consider the questions, record your responses below, and bring them to class.

For activities that will be done in class, as discussions or group activities, it is still beneficial to do some reflection before class to prepare.

1. What interventions are currently in place for this syndrome?

   _____

   _____

   _____

2. Are the interventions consistent with evidence-based practices?

   _____

   _____

   _____

3. Are these interventions addressing the core needs of the resident?

4. Are there any additional assessments or interventions the group would suggest to improve care or reduce risk for further complications related to this syndrome? For example, would additional medication review, specific physical therapy, nutritional support, or a change in monitoring practices be beneficial?

5. How might the nursing team coordinate care to address this syndrome in the context of a long-term care setting?

6. How can other members of the healthcare team (e.g., physician, dietitian, physical therapist) contribute to a more holistic care plan?

7. How does this geriatric syndrome affect the resident's functional status and quality of life?

8. How can nurses advocate for the resident's needs and quality of life by making appropriate interventions?

___

Critical Reflection

At the end of the discussion, your instructor may ask you to write a brief reflection (five to seven sentences) on how this experience impacted your understanding of caring for residents with geriatric syndromes. In your reflection, you should address the following questions:

1. How did the experience change your perspective on geriatric care?
2. What additional nursing skills or knowledge do you need to enhance your ability to care for residents with these conditions?
3. What role do nurses play in advocating for older adults with multiple health challenges?

Use the space below to write your reflection.

___

CHAPTER 7

DEVELOPING THE WORKFORCE OF THE FUTURE

–Maureen Saxon-Gioia, MSHSA, BSN, RN; Christine Mueller, PhD, RN, FGSA, FAAN; Emily Franke, MSW, LSW; Anneliese Perry, MS, NHA, CECM

BRIEF CHAPTER SUMMARY

As you consider your nursing career, it is important to know about the care-delivery models and the professional nursing opportunities in nursing homes. As the name implies, *nursing homes* are intended to provide nursing care to persons who are there for long-term care or transitional/short-term care.

This chapter outlines roles of nursing staff in nursing homes and provides details about the key positions: the director of nursing (DON), licensed nurses (registered nurses [RNs] and licensed practical/vocational nurses [LPNs/LVNs]), unlicensed nursing staff (commonly referred to as certified nursing assistants [CNAs] or nurse aides), and advanced practice RNs.

Some of the key factors that reflect the nurse practice work environment (care-delivery models and metrics for quality of care) are outlined. We explore opportunities for career advancement and professional growth for nurses in nursing homes. The chapter concludes with an overview of two key opportunities to enhance nurse preparation for practice in the nursing home setting: academic-practice partnerships and nurse residency programs.

> **CHAPTER LEARNING OUTCOMES**
> - Describe key roles and positions for nurse staffing and leadership in nursing homes
> - Examine nursing care models, scope, and practices that support collaborative care and professional development in nursing homes
> - Discuss opportunities to enhance nurse preparation for practice in the nursing home setting: academic-practice partnerships and nurse residency programs

DISCUSSION QUESTIONS

Your instructor may use these questions as a group activity and class discussion, so consider the questions, record your responses below, and bring them to class.

For activities that will be done in class, as discussions or group activities, it is still beneficial to do some reflection before class to prepare.

1. Discuss the various benefits of professional nursing practice within the nursing home setting. How do nursing homes provide unique opportunities for RNs to develop specialized skills, enhance their autonomy, and build long-term relationships with residents? Consider the advantages of working in a setting that focuses on gerontological care, as well as the potential for career advancement and leadership development. How do these factors contribute to job satisfaction and overall professional growth for nurses working in long-term care?

    _____

    _____

    _____

    _____

2. Discuss the potential challenges of professional nursing practice in a nursing home setting. Consider factors such as managing complex, chronic health conditions, addressing staffing shortages, navigating regulatory requirements, and providing high-quality care in an environment with limited resources. How do these challenges impact nurse workload, job satisfaction, and the overall quality of care for residents? Additionally, explore the emotional and physical demands of working in long-term care and the potential for burnout among nursing staff.

    _____

    _____

    _____

    _____

3. Discuss how nurses contribute to the interdisciplinary care team in the nursing home setting. How do nurses collaborate with other healthcare professionals—such as physicians, social workers, physical therapists, dietitians, and occupational therapists—to provide holistic, patient-centered care for residents?

   Consider the unique role of nurses in care planning, assessment, and ongoing monitoring of residents' health, as well as their contributions to communication, coordination, and advocacy within the interdisciplinary team.

4. How do nurses' expertise in clinical care, as well as their ability to build relationships with residents and families, enhance the overall quality of care in a long-term care environment? Additionally, explore how nurses act as a bridge between medical, social, and emotional aspects of care in the nursing home.

NEXTGEN NCLEX STYLE QUESTIONS

1. In a long-term care facility, the DON is establishing clinical systems to align nursing practices with various standards. Which of the following is NOT typically within the scope of the DON's responsibilities in this process?

    a. Ensuring practices align with RN and LPN/LVN scopes of practice set by state boards

    b. Implementing evidence-based best practices in geriatric nursing care

    c. Prescribing specific treatment plans for individual residents

    d. Configuring team nursing approaches to optimize all nursing team members' capacities

2. An RN and LPN are working together in a long-term care facility. A new resident with multiple chronic conditions is admitted, requiring a comprehensive care plan. According to their scope of practice, which task is most appropriate for the RN to complete?

    a. Assisting the resident with daily hygiene needs and reporting any skin abnormalities to the physician

    b. Administering prescribed medications to the resident and documenting the administration in the medication record

    c. Performing an initial comprehensive assessment and developing an individualized care plan for the resident

    d. Assisting with wound dressing changes and observing for signs of infection

3. In a nursing home utilizing a professional practice model for care delivery, which action by an RN best demonstrates effective accountability and supports quality care for residents?

    a. Regularly assigning the same nursing assistants to specific residents to promote familiarity

    b. Conducting huddles with the nursing staff to communicate resident observations and changes

    c. Delegating routine assessments to nursing assistants while monitoring their progress

    d. Relying on established care plans to guide decision-making without frequent updates

4. A nursing home has recently implemented a Nurse Residency Program to support new graduate nurses. Which of the following components is essential for ensuring the program's effectiveness in preparing nurse residents for practice in this setting?

    a. Allowing nurse residents to fill staffing shortages during the program

    b. Providing geriatric care competency-based education

    c. Limiting the duration of the program to three months

    d. Focusing solely on technical skills training

5. Which of the following roles of an RN in a nursing home involves using evidence-based assessments and interventions to provide individualized care for residents?

    a. Care role model

    b. Gerontological nurse

    c. Care partner

    d. Mentor

CASE STUDY: Stepping Into Leadership—Exploring the Role of a Director of Nursing in Long-Term Care

This case study focuses on the essential skills and experience required for a director of nursing role in a nursing home. Learners will assess key leadership competencies, explore the interview process, and learn how to evaluate a facility.

Objective

Describe the knowledge, skills, and experience needed by directors of nursing in nursing homes.

Preparation

To prepare for this case study, learners should read/review the following:

- Acello, B. (2020). *The long-term care director of nursing field guide* (4th ed.). HCPro. https://hcmarketplace.com/media/wysiwyg/DONFG4_browse.pdf

- American Organization for Nursing Leadership. (2015). *Nurse executive competencies: Post acute care.* https://www.aonl.org/sites/default/files/aone/nec-post-acute.pdf

- American Organization for Nursing Leadership. (2022). *Nurse leader core competencies.* https://www.aonl.org/system/files/media/file/2024/06/AONL_CCDocument_Pg3Update_060524_PRO.pdf

- Bryant, N., & Stone, R. (2022, March). *Enhancing frontline nurse management in long-term care services and support* [Research brief]. LeadingAge LTSS Center. https://ltsscenter.org/reports/Enhancing_Frontline_Nurse_Management_in_LTSS.pdf

- Fineczko, J., Chu, C., Cranley, L., Wills, A., & McGilton, K. (2023, Nov. 6). Examining the director of nursing role in long-term care: An integrative review. *Journal of Nursing Management.* https://doi.org/10.1155/2023/8200746

- NurseiO. (2022, Oct. 28). *13 essential leadership skills in long-term care facilities.* https://nurseio.com/leadership-skills-in-long-term-care/

- M. U. Sinclair School of Nursing, University of Missouri. (2015). *Observational indicators of nursing home care quality instrument.* https://nursinghomehelp.org/oiq-guide/oiq-instrument-nursing-home-version/

- Saxon-Gioia, M., Franke, E., Siegel, E., Petillo, F., Mueller, C., & Weiss, J. (2024). Developing the workforce of the future. In J. Reifsnyder, A. Kolanowski, & J. Dunbar-Jacobs (Eds), *Practice & Leadership in Nursing Homes: Building on Academic-Practice Partnerships* (pp. 159–181). Sigma Theta Tau International.

Presentation of the Case

Jennifer is an RN who graduated with a BSN degree 10 years ago. She worked in a neuro-surgical unit as a staff and charge nurse for two years and then became the nurse manager for the unit for three years. She has spent the last five years of practice for a large health system's home infusion therapy program, where she served as the director for the program. Jennifer enjoys management and administration and is currently considering a position as a DON in a 120-bed nursing home in her community.

After Jennnifer completed a self-assessment of the knowledge, skills, and experience she had and needed for the position, she determined she wanted to apply for the position. Her application was reviewed favorably, and she was invited to an interview with the administrator of the nursing home.

Questions

Your instructor may use these questions as a group activity and class discussion, so consider the questions, record your responses below, and bring them to class.

For activities that will be done in class, as discussions or group activities, it is still beneficial to do some reflection before class to prepare.

1. To help Jennifer, assess whether this position is the right fit for her. What knowledge, skills, and experience would be needed for this position?

2. To prepare for the interview, what information could she obtain in advance about the nursing home?

3. What questions should she ask the administrator during the interview and why?

4. What things should she look for as she tours the facility during her interview and why?

5. Who else should she ask to meet with during the interview and why?

IN-CLASS ACTIVITIES OR ASSIGNMENTS

Your instructor may assign these as in-class activities or as reflection activities done outside of class, so consider the questions, record your responses below, and bring them to class.

For activities that will be done in class, as discussions or group activities, it is still beneficial to do some reflection before class to prepare.

Assignment: Nurse Leadership—The Director of Nursing (DON) Role in the Nursing Home

This is a class or online assignment that can be done in small groups or individually.

Objectives
- Understand the scope of leadership responsibilities for the DON in a nursing home
- Examine the impact of nursing leadership on resident outcomes and culture of the nursing home
- Explore challenges and problem-solving strategies deployed by DONs

Assignment Instructions

CMS regulations require a DON in all nursing homes. The DON serves as a member of the top leadership team, collaborating with the licensed nursing home administrator and medical director. In this position, the DON oversees all nursing personnel, including associate or assistant DONs, nurse managers, supervisors, and nursing staff who may report directly or indirectly to the DON.

1. Identify a nursing home within your local area. You can search by zip code using the CMS Care Compare website: https://www.medicare.gov/care-compare/?redirect=true&providerType=NursingHome
2. Contact the DON at the identified nursing home to introduce yourself and ask to schedule a time to interview them about their role.
3. Prepare at least seven questions to ask the DON during the interview. Questions should elicit responses related to:
    - Key responsibilities and daily tasks
    - Common challenges experienced
    - Regulatory requirements in the DON role
    - Leadership impact on resident outcomes and culture of the organization
    - Positive benefits of the DON role
4. Conduct the interview and thank the DON for their time.
5. Prepare to discuss what you learned during the interview with the class.
    - Share what surprised you the most about the DON role.
    - Discuss the scope and impact of the leadership role.

Assignment: Nursing Roles Within the Nursing Home Setting

This is a class or online assignment that can be done in small groups or individually.

Objectives

- Research and articulate the essential qualifications, skills, and responsibilities required for a selected nursing role in a nursing home.
- Utilize persuasive language and marketing strategies to effectively highlight the benefits and opportunities of the selected nursing position, aiming to attract qualified candidates by emphasizing aspects such as work environment, career growth, and the impact on resident care.
- Design a visually appealing and professional flyer that effectively communicates the job details, using appropriate layout, fonts, colors, and imagery to capture attention and attract RNs to the role.

Assignment Instructions

As noted in Chapter 7 of the textbook, there are multiple opportunities for career advancement for RNs in nursing homes. These roles are in the areas of nursing administration, infection control and prevention, staff development, quality assurance and improvement, and coordination of assessment and care planning.

1. Select one role of the RNs in the nursing home from the section "Roles and Career Advancement Opportunities for RNs in Nursing Homes" in Chapter 7 to research.

2. Identify the qualifications, skills, responsibilities, and pertinent nursing home regulations for the selected role. Federal nursing home regulations can be found in Title 42, Part 483 of the *Code of Federal Regulations*. These regulations are accessible through the U.S. Government Publishing Office at ecfr.gov.

3. Utilizing the information you gathered during your research, design a flyer to highlight the benefits and opportunities of the selected role. Use persuasive language to emphasize the impact of the role in the nursing home. The flyer should include:

    - RN role: Clearly state the role selected.
    - Qualifications: List the essential qualifications (e.g., licensure, experience, certifications).
    - Responsibilities: Summarize the key responsibilities of the role.
    - Benefits: Highlight the benefits of the role.

4. Get creative! Choose a layout that will stand out and appeal to potential applicants. Consider using software like Canva, Adobe Spark, or Microsoft Publisher to create the flyer.

Optional Activities

1. Students may display their flyers in the classroom and discuss the variety of options available in the nursing home setting.

2. Display the flyers around the classroom. Allow students the option to view all flyers. Ask students to identify:

    a. The most persuasive flyer

    b. The job that appeals the most to them after reading the descriptions and benefits

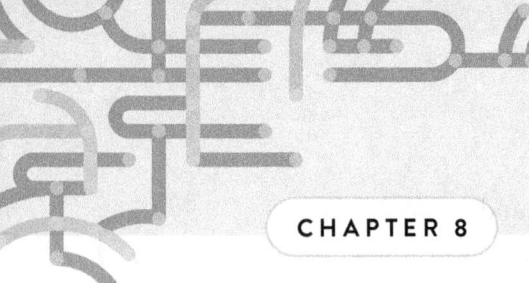

CHAPTER 8

STAFF DEVELOPMENT AND TRAINING

–Andrea Sillner, PhD, RN, GCNS-BC; Sophie Campbell, MSN, RN, CRRN, RAC-CT, CNDLTC

BRIEF CHAPTER SUMMARY

Staff development and training in nursing homes are essential to ensuring high-quality care and improving patient outcomes (American Health Care Association, 2023). Training programs target a variety of staff roles, including nurses, nursing assistants, and support staff, focusing on areas such as clinical skills, dementia care, infection control, and person-centered practices (National Hartford Center of Gerontological Nursing Excellence, 2023). Effective staff training can enhance job satisfaction, reduce turnover, and foster a positive workplace culture (Revisiting Teaching Nursing Home Project, 2023). Additionally, addressing the self-care needs of nursing home staff is crucial, as high stress and burnout rates among caregivers can negatively impact both staff well-being and patient care (National Institute on Aging, 2023). By offering ongoing professional development, promoting self-care practices, and providing supportive work environments, nursing homes can enhance care quality and staff retention (NYU Hartford Institute for Geriatric Nursing, 2023).

> **CHAPTER LEARNING OUTCOMES**
> - Describe staff training and development in the context of the nursing home environment
> - Explain the importance and elements of staff performance evaluation
> - List methods for staff training and development

DISCUSSION QUESTIONS

Your instructor may use these questions as a group activity and class discussion, so consider the questions, record your responses below, and bring them to class.

For activities that will be done in class, as discussions or group activities, it is still beneficial to do some reflection before class to prepare.

1. In nursing homes, the organizational structure and nursing hierarchy play a critical role in ensuring effective care delivery and staff collaboration. Based on your clinical experience or understanding of nursing home settings, describe the typical nursing hierarchy and the roles of different nursing staff (e.g., RN, LPN, CNA, and others). Also consider the RN or LPN Nurse Supervisor and Manager.

2. How does the role of each nursing staff member contribute to resident outcomes?

3. How does this hierarchy impact the flow of communication, decision-making, and overall nursing home resident care?

4. Additionally, in your opinion, what are the potential challenges or benefits of the current hierarchical structure in a nursing home setting (where you provide care or have had a clinical experience)?

5. How might changes to the organizational structure or nursing hierarchy improve staff teamwork and care quality?

___

___

___

___

Additional Discussion Question: Relevance of Coaching and Training in The Nursing Home

Note: This question could be assigned by your facilitator as part of a discussion board assignment or as a written assignment since it is more complex than the general discussion questions above.

In nursing homes, the nursing staff are essential to resident care delivery including quality of care, quality of life and safety. Often staff have been in their positions for several years or they are very new to their roles in nursing. Based on your clinical experience or understanding of nursing home settings, discuss the importance of coaching and training for the nursing team members. Also consider the potential negative impact of not providing relevant, adequate training and coaching for nursing team members.

How does training and coaching positively impact retention of nursing team members? How does training and coaching ensure quality of care, quality of life and safety for nursing home residents and nursing team members? What are challenges to ensure that coaching and training are provided and are relevant, adequate, and useful? How does training and coaching ensure that nursing team members feel valued and invested in?

Consider aspects such as:

- How does training ensure competency in care delivery to ensure quality of care and resident safety?
- Does training assist only the new nursing team members/
- What are your ideas for how frequently training should be delivered to direct caregivers and nursing team members based on the time constraints of delivering resident care and having staff on all shifts
- How might coaching and training assist nursing team members to feel the organization is investing in them and valuing their contribution to the organization?
- Are there ways to provide coaching that is effective and fun while ensuring team members are heard and their concerns are acted upon?

NEXTGEN NCLEX STYLE QUESTIONS

1. A nurse working in a nursing home is experiencing increasing levels of stress and burnout due to a heavy workload, high resident acuity, and limited support. The nurse is concerned about the impact this might have on their ability to provide quality care. Which of the following actions should the nurse prioritize to prevent burnout and maintain professional competency?

    a. Work extra shifts to help with staffing shortages and provide support to the team

    b. Seek out professional development opportunities and relaxation techniques

    c. Take time off to recover but avoid discussing stress with colleagues

    d. Focus on completing tasks quickly to meet performance expectations

2. A nurse is tasked with assessing a newly admitted resident in a long-term care facility. The nurse is certified in geriatric nursing and has experience with dementia care. What is the most important aspect of the nurse's role during the admission process to ensure high-quality care for the resident?

    a. Focus primarily on completing administrative paperwork to meet facility requirements

    b. Evaluate the resident's medical history to determine a treatment plan

    c. Establish a therapeutic relationship to assess the resident's physical and emotional needs

    d. Assign primary caregiving responsibilities to a nursing assistant

3. A nurse working in a nursing home has noticed a high turnover rate among nursing assistants. Many of the assistants are reporting feelings of being overwhelmed and unsupported in their roles. Which of the following actions should the nurse take to address the burnout among nursing assistants?

    a. Offer regular debriefing sessions and encourage open communication about work stress

    b. Advise the nursing assistants to focus on completing their tasks more efficiently

    c. Allow the nursing assistants to take longer breaks without altering their workload

    d. Reduce resident care responsibilities to give nursing assistants more downtime

4. A nurse who passed state boards in the past year and had been working at the hospital has transferred to the nursing home. The new nurse observes an experienced senior nurse not following infection prevention and control standards of practice during completion of a wound treatment. How should the new nurse address the situation to ensure high-quality care for the resident?

a. Tell the experienced senior nurse that she will complete the wound treatment to ensure infection prevention and control standards of practice are followed.

b. Report the experienced and senior nurses practices to the director of nursing, infection preventionist, and compliance officer

c. Discuss the standards of practice for infection prevention and control related to wound treatments with the senior and experienced nurse and share ideas and methods with her so they can ensure quality and safe care for this resident and other residents

d. Immediately turn in her resignation to prevent being associated with a possible resident nosocomial facility acquired infection while she was completing orientation

5. A nurse working in a long-term care facility notices they are frequently feeling fatigued and emotionally drained at the end of each shift. Despite having a passion for geriatric nursing, they are beginning to doubt their ability to continue in their role. Which of the following strategies should the nurse implement to improve their well-being and manage work-related stress?

    a. Reduce interactions with residents to minimize emotional involvement

    b. Take on additional shifts to overcome feelings of inadequacy

    c. Focus only on the physical needs of residents, ignoring emotional care

    d. Participate in mindfulness exercises and seek support from a mentor or counselor

CASE STUDY: Nurse Burnout in a Nursing Home Setting

Background Information

Nurse Demographics

Name: Sarah Thompson, RN

Age: 38 years

Years of experience: 12 years

Current role: Charge nurse on a dementia unit at within Brookstone Care Center nursing home

Certification: Certified in geriatric nursing and dementia care

Family: Married with two young children (ages 5 and 8)

Work hours: Full time, 40 hours/week with rotating shifts, including nights and weekends

Length of employment at the facility: Six years

Nursing Home Environment

Facility: Brookstone Care Center, a 120-bed nursing home located in a suburban area

Unit: Sarah works on the Memory Care Unit, which primarily serves residents with Alzheimer's disease and other dementias. The unit has 25 beds, and each nurse is responsible for up to 15 residents during their shift.

Staffing issues: Brookstone Care Center has been struggling with high staff turnover, particularly among nursing assistants and RNs. The facility has been unable to hire enough staff to cover shifts, leading to frequent overtime and use of contracted staff, especially during the night shifts.

Work environment: The facility is in a constant state of flux, with frequent staffing changes. Many of Sarah's colleagues are also experiencing burnout and express frustration with the constant demands of the job. The residents often exhibit challenging behaviors, such as aggression, wandering, and agitation, which require specialized care and patience.

Management support: The facility's management is aware of staffing issues but has limited resources to address them. Sarah and her colleagues have voiced concerns about burnout, but management has only implemented short-term solutions, such as offering overtime shifts, bonuses, use of contracted agency staff, and providing basic inservice training on managing dementia-related behaviors.

Presentation of the Case

Sarah Thompson, a dedicated RN, has worked at Brookstone Care Center for six years. She has always been passionate about caring for the elderly and finds great satisfaction in her role on the Memory Care Unit, where she can make a difference in the lives of residents with dementia. However, in recent months, Sarah has started to feel overwhelmed and exhausted.

Sarah's work-life balance has become increasingly difficult to manage. At home, she is responsible for her two young children, and her spouse works long hours, often leaving Sarah to manage the home and children on her own. The demands of her family life, combined with her often greater than 40-hour workweek, are taking a toll on her physical and emotional well-being. She has also been picking up extra shifts to cover the unit's staffing needs, leading to increased fatigue and reduced time for rest.

At work, Sarah is regularly faced with high levels of stress. The Memory Care Unit frequently experiences aggressive and agitated behaviors from residents, which require continuous intervention and specialized care. Sarah's unit is often facing staffing challenges, with one additional licensed staff and two nursing assistants to provide care for 25 memory support residents. Sarah finds herself constantly rushing between tasks, such as assisting with feeding, administering medications, monitoring vital signs, and addressing challenging behaviors, while trying to ensure a safe and dignified environment for her residents and maintain the skills of the care team members on the unit.

The nursing assistants on her unit, many of whom are new to dementia care, often need extra guidance, and Sarah feels the responsibility of teaching them while managing her own workload. The constant demands are leaving her emotionally drained. Over the past few weeks, she has noticed that she feels disconnected from her residents and has been experiencing feelings of inadequacy as a nurse and a caregiver. Her coworkers express similar frustrations, and morale on the unit is low. Several staff members have voiced concerns about the lack of management support and the high turnover rate among nursing assistants.

Sarah has always been committed to her profession and prided herself on being able to care for others, but now she is feeling increasingly disconnected and exhausted. She is beginning to question her ability to continue in her role and is struggling with the emotional weight of her job.

Questions

Your instructor may use these questions as a group activity and class discussion, so consider the questions, record your responses below, and bring them to class.

For activities that will be done in class, as discussions or group activities, it is still beneficial to do some reflection before class to prepare.

1. What factors do you think are contributing to Sarah's burnout?

2. How might Sarah's colleagues be experiencing burnout, and how can this affect resident care?

3. What strategies can the nursing home's management implement to address burnout and improve staff well-being?

4. What self-care strategies can Sarah implement to help prevent further burnout?

5. How can the nursing team create a supportive work environment to prevent burnout?

Conclusion

Burnout is a common and serious issue for healthcare workers, particularly those in high-stress environments such as nursing homes. By addressing staffing challenges, offering support, providing coaching and training when needed and when requested, and implementing self-care practices, organizations can minimize the risk of burnout and improve the well-being of their staff. It is crucial to create a supportive work environment where both management and staff work together to ensure high-quality care for residents while maintaining staff health and morale.

IN-CLASS ACTIVITIES OR ASSIGNMENTS

Your instructor may assign these as in-class activities or as reflection activities done outside of class.

For activities that will be done in class, as discussions or group activities, it is still beneficial to do some reflection before class to prepare.

Group Activity: Identifying Roles and Educational Preparation of Nursing Staff in the Nursing Home

This activity may be assigned by your instructor as an in-person activity, a discussion board online, or used as a post-clinical conference discussion.

Objectives

- Identify and describe the key roles of nursing care staff in the nursing home setting
- Understand the educational preparation and responsibilities associated with each role

Materials needed: Handout "Roles & Responsibilities Overview" listing and describing common provider roles in a nursing home

Handout: Roles & Responsibilities Overview

1. Registered nurse (RN)

   Key responsibilities: RNs oversee the care of residents, develop care plans, administer medications, and coordinate with other healthcare professionals. They perform assessments, monitor for changes in the residents' health status, and provide treatments as prescribed by physicians. RNs supervise and oversee LPNs and CNAs.

   Educational preparation: Must have a bachelor of science in nursing (BSN), associate degree in nursing (ADN), or a diploma in nursing. Must pass the NCLEX-RN exam to become licensed.

   Continuing education may be required for licensure renewal, particularly in specialized areas like geriatric care.

   Certifications: Advanced certifications may include certified geriatric nurse or certified dementia practitioner.

2. Licensed practical nurse (LPN)

   Key responsibilities: LPNs work under the supervision and oversight of RNs. They administer medications and treatments, monitor vital signs, provide basic nursing care, assist with activities of daily living (ADLs), and report changes in the resident's condition to RNs or physicians. They are required to document in the medical records what they have evaluated in resident care and medication and treatment administration. LNs fill the majority of the licensed nurse positions in nursing homes.

Educational preparation: Must complete a practical nursing program (usually one year in length) at an accredited and state approved LPN training program, which requires students to possess either a high school diploma or a GED. In some cases, they will accept high school students. Must pass the NCLEX-PN exam to become licensed.

Continuing education may be required for licensure renewal.

Certifications: LPNs may specialize in areas like IV therapy, geriatric care, or wound care through additional training and certification. LPNs must adhere to state practice acts regarding their practice level.

3. Certified nursing assistant (CNA)

    Key responsibilities: CNAs assist residents with Activities of Daily Living, such as bathing, dressing, feeding, and toileting. They monitor residents for changes in condition, assist with functional mobility and self-care, and report observations to nursing staff. They provide hands-on, direct care and are often the primary contact for residents and families. They document the level of assistance they have provided and often they provide or assist with Restorative Nursing Program treatment services to attain and/or maintain functional mobility and self-care.

    Educational preparation: CNAs must complete a state-approved training program (typically 4–12 weeks) that includes classroom instruction and clinical practice. After completing the program, they must pass a state competency exam to be certified.

    Certifications: CNA certification is required for employment in nursing homes, and certification must be renewed periodically (usually every one to two years), which may involve continuing education. Regulations also require a specific number of hours of education each year and each nursing home must ensure the CNAs are sufficiently educated and trained to provide the care required for the residents in the facility.

4. Feeding assistant/aide:

    Key responsibilities: Feeding assistants help residents with meals, ensuring they are able to eat at the highest level of independence for safety or with assistance. They may provide hand-over-hand assistance to residents who have difficulty feeding themselves, help residents with eating, and assist in ensuring safety during meals (e.g., avoiding choking hazards and aspiration).

    Educational preparation: Typically requires on-the-job training or completion of a short, specialized feeding assistant program, which often takes about one to two days.

    Certification: In some states, feeding assistants must be state-certified, which requires completing a course and passing an exam. This is generally a basic certification for safe feeding practices in the nursing home.

5. Medication aide:

    Key responsibilities: Medication aides are responsible for administering routine medications to residents under the supervision of an RN or LPN. They must document medication administration, and may be asked to monitor for side effects, and report any issues related to medications to nursing staff.

Educational preparation: Medication aides must complete a state-approved medication aide training program (usually about 100–120 hours of training, including both classroom and clinical practice). They must pass a state competency exam and meet continuing education requirements for certification renewal.

Certifications: Medication aides must be certified in the state where they work, and certification must be renewed periodically.

Activity Steps

1. Your instructor will lead an in-class group activity to explore the roles and responsibilities of care staff in a nursing home. Learners will discuss and identify what each role entails and what the primary responsibilities are for each. They should write down their findings.

2. Each group will then present their findings to the class, describing:
   - What each role does in the nursing home
   - The level of education and training required for each role
   - Any certifications or licensure necessary
   - Scope of practice (how do the roles overlap or complement one another in the care?)

Class Discussion

After the group presentations, the facilitator will lead a class-wide discussion on the following points. Use the space below to record your notes.

1. What do you think are the most important qualifications for each role?

   _____
   _____
   _____
   _____

2. How do these roles work together to ensure optimal resident care in a nursing home?

   _____
   _____
   _____
   _____

3. What might happen if any of these roles were not filled or inadequately prepared?

4. What additional certifications or training might benefit staff working in a nursing home?

5. What additional training and coaching might benefit nursing staff at each level working in a nursing home?

6. How could the nursing home provide ongoing education and support for staff to reduce burnout and improve care delivery?

Suggested Learning Reflection

Learners should individually reflect on what they've learned about the roles and educational preparation of nursing home staff. Write down one strategy or idea you could apply to improve care and teamwork in a nursing home setting, based on the discussion. Use the space below for your reflection.

_____

_____

_____

Conclusion

This activity helps learners recognize the various roles in nursing homes, their educational preparation, and the importance of each role in providing high-quality care. By understanding these roles and their scope of practice, learners can appreciate the importance of collaboration, ongoing education, and adequate training to maintain a high standard of care and prevent burnout in nursing homes.

Learning Activity: Exploring Methods for Nursing Home Nursing Staff Training and Development

This assignment may be done in class as a group activity and discussion or assigned as an individual project.

Objectives

- Identify various methods for training and development of nursing staff in nursing homes
- Explore online resources and assess their effectiveness
- Recommend strategies for continuous professional development in long-term care settings

Assignment Instructions

Step 1: Research Online Resources

In this first step, learners will individually or in small groups research online resources related to training and development opportunities for nursing staff in nursing homes.

Each group or individual should list at least three to five online resources that provide training and development opportunities, specifically for nursing staff in nursing homes.

Step 2: Identify Training Methods

After researching the online resources, learners should list different methods for training and developing nursing home staff.

Step 3: Assess the Effectiveness of the Resources and Methods

In small groups or individually, learners should discuss or write about the effectiveness of each training method and resource identified. They should consider the following:

- **Accessibility:** Is the resource easy to access? Does it require travel, or can it be done online?
- **Flexibility:** Does the training accommodate different schedules and staff needs (e.g., for night shift workers)?
- **Relevance:** How applicable is the training content to nursing home practice, especially in the context of challenges like dementia care, managing behaviors, and infection control?
- **Engagement:** Is the resource engaging enough to keep staff interested and invested in the learning process? Does it include interactive elements?
- **Outcomes:** Are there measurable outcomes (e.g., certifications, improved care practices) associated with these training methods?

Step 4: Share Findings and Develop Recommendations

In a group or individual presentation or class discussion, learners will present their findings and propose strategies for improving nursing staff training in nursing homes based on the resources and methods explored. Some guiding questions to address:

1. Which training methods would be most effective in a nursing home setting, and why?
2. Which training methods would be most effective for each of the levels of nursing team members in the nursing home and why?
3. How can online resources be integrated into regular nursing home staff schedules?
4. What do you believe is the most effective method of training if team members have limited time for training?
5. What are the benefits of continuous training and development for nursing staff in nursing homes?
6. What role does leadership play in ensuring that staff are continuously trained and supported?
7. What is an effective response to nursing leadership who believe that there is no time in the schedule or opportunity for nursing team members to attend education?
8. What is the best method to share education and information obtained in external education with team members for maximal benefit from the education?

Reflection Questions

Your instructor may use these questions as a group activity and class discussion, so consider the questions, record your responses below, and bring them to class.

For activities that will be done in class, as discussions or group activities, it is still beneficial to do some reflection before class to prepare.

1. Which training method do you believe is most important for nursing home staff? Why?

   _____
   _____
   _____
   _____

2. How can nursing homes ensure that staff members stay up to date with the latest best practices in geriatric care?

   _____
   _____
   _____
   _____

3. How can nursing homes remain compliant with federal and state regulatory requirements for staff education?

   _____
   _____
   _____
   _____

4. What is the most effective method to ensure nursing staff are sufficiently educated to deliver the care required by a changing level of acuity in the nursing home?

5. What challenges might a nursing home face when implementing continuous training programs for its staff, and how could they overcome these challenges?

6. How does ongoing professional development contribute to preventing staff burnout and improving resident care quality?

Conclusion

This learning activity helps learners explore various methods for training and developing nursing home staff, emphasizing the importance of continuous education and professional growth. By identifying and evaluating online resources and training methods, learners can suggest actionable strategies to improve nursing staff skills, foster engagement, and enhance care delivery in nursing homes.

APPLICATION OF CONTENT IN THE CLINICAL AND/OR SIMULATION SETTING: Nursing Home Staff Performance Evaluation

Simulation & Role-Play Activity

Your instructor will lead an in-class role-playing activity to explore possible responses to the scenario.

By the end of this simulation, learners will understand the importance of staff performance evaluations in a nursing home setting. They will practice conducting a staff evaluation meeting between an RN and an RN Manager or Director of Nursing (DON). Learners will identify key elements in a performance evaluation, including communication, goal-setting, feedback, and addressing areas for improvement.

Scenario: The meeting takes place in the DON's office. Sarah Thompson is scheduled for a midyear performance review, and Lisa Harris, the DON, is responsible for conducting the evaluation.

The goal of the meeting is to discuss Sarah's performance, address any strengths or areas for improvement, set goals, and provide feedback. Both parties should focus on open communication and creating an action plan for ongoing professional development.

Roles:

1. **RN:** Sarah Thompson, RN, a charge nurse on the Memory Care Unit, has been working at the facility for six years. Sarah has been performing well overall but is experiencing some difficulty managing her workload due to the understaffing on the unit. Her performance review is coming up, and she needs to discuss some challenges she has been facing, as well as her achievements.

2. **RN manager/DON:** Lisa Harris, RN, the Director of Nursing at Brookstone Care Center, is conducting Sarah's performance evaluation. She is tasked with evaluating Sarah's performance. Lisa will focus on recognizing her strengths (e.g., resident care, teamwork) but also address areas where there is room for improvement (e.g., managing stress, delegation). She will also need to set some specific goals for Sarah's ongoing development.

3. **Nursing team members working with Sarah:** You are tasked with responding to the manager/DON regarding the performance of Sarah in her role with general comments and specific comments (this should be a standard of practice for collecting information about performance prior to the evaluations from the team members working with the team member being evaluated).

Debriefing Questions

Your instructor will ask students to reflect on their experience during the role-play. Your instructor may use the following questions as a group activity and class discussion, so consider the questions, record your responses below, and bring them to class.

For activities that will be done in class, as discussions or group activities, it is still beneficial to do some reflection before class to prepare.

1. What went well in the performance evaluation?

2. What are the challenges you encountered when discussing areas for improvement? How were they addressed?

3. How can effective performance evaluations contribute to staff retention and overall job satisfaction in nursing homes?

4. What strategies can the RN Manager/DON use to ensure that feedback is received positively and leads to positive change?

5. How might the RN Manager/DON further support staff who are struggling with workload or burnout?

_____

_____

_____

_____

Clinical Activity or Assignment: Identifying and Addressing Burnout/Stress in Nursing Home Staff

This activity could be assigned by your instructor as a post-clinical group discussion, a discussion board topic, or an individual written assignment.

Instructions

Reflecting on your clinical experience in the nursing home, identify any potential causes of burnout and stress that you observed among the nursing staff. Consider factors such as workload, staffing levels, resident care demands, and emotional challenges. Also consider factors such as not having the education to perform the care that residents require and none of the leadership staff or other staff are able to assist with training. Additionally, consider factors such as not feeling invested in or valued by the nursing home or nursing leadership. What symptoms of burnout or stress did you notice in the staff, and how did this impact their ability to provide care?

Based on your observations, propose strategies or interventions that could help minimize burnout and stress for nursing home staff. Think about both organizational-level changes and individual self-care practices that could improve the work environment and the well-being of the staff.

REFERENCES

American Health Care Association. (2023). *Education.* https://www.ahcancal.org/education/Pages/default.aspx

National Hartford Center of Gerontological Nursing Excellence. (2023). *Staff development in geriatric nursing.* https://www.ahcancal.org/Research/Innovation/Pages/Workforce.aspx

National Institute on Aging. (2023). *Training and career development.* https://www.nia.nih.gov/research/training

NYU Hartford Institute for Geriatric Nursing. (2023). *Online education.* https://hign.org/consultgeri-resources/online-education

Revisiting Teaching Nursing Home Project. (2023). *Improving nursing home care through education.* https://www.nursing.umaryland.edu/rtnh/

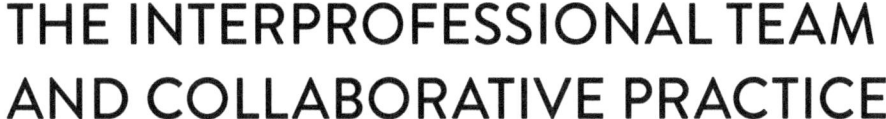

CHAPTER 9

THE INTERPROFESSIONAL TEAM AND COLLABORATIVE PRACTICE

–Andrea Sillner, PhD, RN, GCNS-BC; Jennifer Sidelinker, DPT, PT;
Anne Bradley Mitchell, PhD, CRNP, FGSA: Michele Orzehoski, DNP, MSN, RN-BC

BRIEF CHAPTER SUMMARY

The interprofessional care team in the nursing home setting is important in delivering high-quality, person-centered care to complex residents. Each member of the interprofessional care team brings a specialized set of skills to the table. The interprofessional team members in a nursing home often include the nurse, pharmacist, physical therapist, occupational therapist, speech therapist, registered dietician, recreation therapist, and social worker.

CHAPTER LEARNING OUTCOMES
- Describe principles of interprofessional practice in the nursing home setting
- Differentiate specialized areas of practice for each team member
- Apply an interprofessional practice model to the care of a resident with complex chronic illness

DISCUSSION QUESTION

Your instructor may use this question as a group activity and class discussion, so consider the question, record your response below, and bring it to class.

Objective: To explore the collaborative roles of interprofessional teams in assessing, discussing, and applying findings related to the 4Ms (What Matters, Medication, Mentation, and Mobility) in the context of nursing home care, and to emphasize the importance of a coordinated approach to ensure optimal resident outcomes (Institute for Healthcare Improvement, 2020).

Question: How do interprofessional teams in nursing homes collaborate to assess, communicate, and apply findings related to the 4Ms?

_____

_____

_____

_____

NEXTGEN NCLEX STYLE QUESTIONS

1. A patient in a nursing home has a history of falls. The nurse, physical therapist, occupational therapist, and social worker are all involved in the resident's care. Which of the following is the most effective way to ensure a coordinated approach to fall prevention?

    a. The nurse develops a comprehensive fall prevention plan and shares it with the other team members.

    b. Each team member independently assesses the resident's risk factors and implements their own interventions.

    c. Each team member conducts a discipline specific assessment, then the team holds a meeting to discuss the resident's case and collaboratively develop a fall prevention and management plan.

    d. The social worker coordinates the team's efforts and ensures that all interventions are implemented consistently.

2. A nursing home resident has a complex medical history, including diabetes, hypertension, and heart failure. The nurse, physician, pharmacist, and dietician are all involved in their care. Which of the following is the best strategy to ensure that the resident's medications are administered correctly and safely?

    a. The nurse administers all medications independently and documents the administration in the electronic medical record.

    b. The pharmacist reviews the patient's medication regimen and discusses the recommendation plan with the nurse.

    c. The physician writes all medication orders, and the nurse administers them as prescribed.

    d. The dietician ensures that the patient's diet is compatible with their medications.

3. A nursing home resident has recently experienced a stroke and is struggling with communication. The nurse, speech therapist, and occupational therapist are all involved in the patient's care. Which of the following is the most effective way to facilitate communication about the resident's plan of care?

    a. The nurse provides one-on-one communication therapy with the resident.

    b. The speech therapist develops a communication plan and provides therapy to the resident.

    c. The occupational therapist focuses on helping the resident regain fine motor skills for writing.

    d. The team collaborates with the patient to develop solutions that improve communication.

4. A resident in the nursing home setting is nearing the end of life. The nurse, physician, social worker, and chaplain are all involved in the patient's care. Which of the following is the best way to ensure that the resident's wishes regarding end-of-life care are respected?

   a. The nurse discusses the What Matters section of the 4Ms with the family and documents them in the electronic health record.

   b. The physician develops a plan of care that is consistent with the resident's preferences and goals.

   c. The social worker facilitates family meetings and provides emotional support to the resident and family.

   d. The team collaborates to develop an individualized plan of care that addresses the resident's physical, emotional, and spiritual needs.

5. A resident in the nursing home has recently been diagnosed with dementia. The nurse, physician, occupational therapist, speech therapist, and social worker are all involved in their care. Which of the following is the most effective way to support quality of life for this resident?

   a. The collaborative interprofessional team works to create a supportive environment that promotes the resident's well-being and quality of life as defined by the resident and their family.

   b. The nurse provides one-on-one care to the resident and ensures that their needs are met.

   c. The physician prescribes medications to manage the resident's behavioral and psychological symptoms of dementia.

   d. The occupational therapist assists the resident with activities of daily living.

CASE STUDY: Interprofessional Team Collaboration

Patient Profile

Name: Mr. Russell Thomas

Age: 84 years

Admission type: Direct admission from home after family difficulties managing his care

Mr. Russell Thomas was initially admitted to the nursing home following a hip fracture from a fall a few months ago. He underwent short-term rehabilitation and made significant progress, eventually returning home. Recently, his family has struggled to assist him with activities of daily living (ADLs), leading to the decision to pursue a direct admission back to the nursing home.

Medical diagnoses:

- Type 2 diabetes: Requires careful monitoring of blood sugar levels and dietary management
- Chronic urinary incontinence: Leads to potential skin integrity issues and requires management strategies
- Progressive dysphagia: Difficulty swallowing, particularly pills, complicates medication administration and nutritional intake
- Recent diagnosis of dementia: Exhibits short-term memory impairment, affecting his ability to remember care routines and recognize family members

Physical assessment:

- Mobility: Exhibits limited mobility, requiring a wheeled walker for ambulation short distances. He demonstrates an unsteady gait, indicative of his previous hip fracture. He also has a very high fall risk.
- Strength: Reduced muscle strength in the lower extremities, likely due to inactivity and the effects of aging
- Cognitive status: Alert but disoriented to time; struggles to recall recent events and personal history
- Nutritional status: Weight loss noted due to difficulties with swallowing and reduced oral intake

Occupational/social/leisure activities:

- Occupational engagement: Mr. Thomas enjoyed gardening and playing card games prior to his fall. He was previously a barber. He is a widower and misses his wife who died 20 years ago. He has expressed frustration over his inability to participate in these activities.
- Social interaction: He is supported by his daughter who lives nearby and is a healthcare professional familiar with the nursing home setting. Otherwise, he has limited interaction with family and friends due to cognitive decline and mobility issues, leading to feelings of isolation.
- Leisure activities: Mr. Thomas previously enjoyed reading the newspaper and watching sports but now struggles to focus and engage in these activities due to his cognitive impairments. He likes sitting outside. He is not a fan of structured activities or groups.

Interprofessional Team Collaboration

Upon Mr. Thomas's admission, an interprofessional team convenes to develop a comprehensive care plan tailored to his needs. The team includes:

1. **Nurse:** Conducts a thorough assessment and monitors Mr. Thomas's medical conditions, ensuring regular blood sugar checks and managing incontinence care to prevent skin breakdown. Documentation of "What Matters" during initial and subsequent assessments. Facilitates recommendations from pharmacy and therapy teams to integrate into plan of care. Fall precautions were also implemented per nursing home protocol.

2. **Pharmacist:** Reviews Mr. Thomas's medication regimen, addressing his difficulty swallowing pills by suggesting alternatives, such as liquid formulations or crushing pills when appropriate. Provides recommendations to the nursing team for medication administration and deprescribing as appropriate.

3. **Physical therapist:** Evaluates Mr. Thomas's mobility and develops a personalized exercise program to improve strength and balance, and a regular restorative ambulation program to enhance his independence and reduce fall risk.

4. **Occupational therapist:** Works with Mr. Thomas to identify adaptive strategies and assistive devices to facilitate ADLs, focusing on improving his ability to engage in meaningful activities such as gardening and card games.

5. **Speech therapist:** Assesses Mr. Thomas's swallowing abilities and implements a tailored plan to address his dysphagia, including dietary modifications (e.g., thickened liquids) and exercises to strengthen swallowing muscles.

6. **Recreation therapist:** Develops a structured program of leisure activities that accommodates Mr. Thomas's interests and abilities, facilitating social interaction and enhancing his quality of life.

7. **Social worker:** Engages with Mr. Thomas and his family to provide emotional support, counseling, and resources for navigating care options. Facilitates family meetings to address concerns and foster communication among team members.

Conclusion

Through coordinated efforts, the interprofessional team will help to ensure that Mr. Thomas receives holistic care tailored to his medical and psychosocial needs. Regular team meetings promote communication and adjustments to the care plan as his condition evolves, aiming to improve his quality of life and support his family during this challenging time.

Questions

Your instructor may use these questions as a group activity and class discussion, so consider the questions, record your responses below, and bring them to class.

For activities that will be done in class, as discussions or group activities, it is still beneficial to do some reflection before class to prepare.

1. **Assessment and care planning:** What specific assessment tools and methods could the nursing team use to evaluate Mr. Thomas's mobility and cognitive function upon admission? How can these assessments inform the development of his individualized care plan?

2. **Medication management:** Considering Mr. Thomas's difficulty swallowing pills, what strategies can the pharmacist implement to ensure he receives his medications safely and effectively? What role should the nursing staff play in monitoring his medication adherence?

3. **Interprofessional communication:** How can the interprofessional team enhance communication and collaboration to ensure that all members are informed about Mr. Thomas's progress and changes in his condition? What strategies can be implemented to facilitate ongoing dialogue among team members?

4. **Family involvement:** In what ways can the social worker engage Mr. Thomas's family in his care plan to better support their emotional needs and address their concerns? What resources or support groups might be beneficial for them?

5. **Activity engagement:** How can the recreation therapist tailor activities to accommodate Mr. Thomas's cognitive impairments while still encouraging participation in social and leisure activities? What adaptive strategies might be effective in helping him reconnect with his interests?

IN-CLASS ACTIVITIES OR ASSIGNMENTS

Your instructor may assign these as in-class activities or as reflection activities done outside of class.

For activities that will be done in class, as discussions or group activities, it is still beneficial to do some reflection before class to prepare.

Learning Activity: Creating a Teaching Resource for Nursing Home Residents and Families

This assignment may be done in class as a group and then discussion or assigned as an individual project.

Objectives

- Educate nursing home residents and their families about the interprofessional roles they will encounter in the nursing home setting
- Enhance understanding of individual team member roles and communication among team members

Materials needed:
- Paper (for pamphlets, flyers, or brochures)
- Markers, colored pencils, or pens
- Access to a computer and printer (optional)
- Example pamphlets or brochures for inspiration
- Reference materials on interprofessional roles (if needed)

Assignment Instructions

1. Your instructor will begin with a brief discussion on the importance of understanding the various interprofessional roles within a nursing home.

2. Your instructor will divide learners into small groups, assigning each group one or two interprofessional roles (e.g., nurse, pharmacist, physical therapist, occupational therapist, speech therapist, recreation therapist, social worker). Each group should research their assigned roles, focusing on:
    - Key responsibilities and functions
    - How the role contributes to resident care
    - Ways the role interacts with residents and families

3. Resource creation: Using your research, each group will create a teaching resource in the form of a pamphlet, flyer, or mini brochure. The resource should include:
    - A clear title (e.g., "Meet Your Care Team: Understanding Interprofessional Roles in Our Nursing Home")
    - A brief description of each role (one to two sentences)
    - Visual elements (images, icons, or diagrams) to enhance engagement
    - Contact information for residents or families to reach out with questions or concerns
    - Tips for how residents and families can engage with each team member effectively

4. Presentation: Each group will present their teaching resource to the class, explaining the roles they covered and how the resources can benefit residents and their families.

5. Feedback: After each presentation, the instructor will facilitate feedback from peers, discussing what was effective and what could be improved.

Suggested Learning Reflection

Reflect on what you learned in the activity about the importance of interprofessional collaboration and effective communication in enhancing the quality of care for residents. Write down one strategy or idea you could apply to improve interprofessional care and teamwork in a nursing home setting. Use the space below for your reflection.

_____

_____

_____

_____

Assignment: Interprofessional Role Exploration

This assignment may be assigned as an individual or small group activity with the option of in-class presentations and/or discussion.

Objectives

- Enhance learners' understanding of the diverse roles within the interprofessional team in a nursing home setting
- Emphasize the importance of collaboration among these professionals in providing high-quality patient care

Instructions

Find a role description for an interprofessional role in the nursing home setting. This could be a role you have encountered during clinical or work experience, or you can choose a role you are interested in learning more about.

Once you have found a role description, research the role and answer the following questions in a short, written response.

1. **Core responsibilities:** What are the primary duties and responsibilities of this role?
2. **Interprofessional collaboration:** What other healthcare professionals commonly collaborate with a person in this role in the nursing home setting?
3. **Unique challenges:** What are some of the unique challenges or obstacles that professionals in this role may face?
4. **Impact on patient care:** How does this role contribute to the overall quality of patient care in the nursing home?

Use the space below for your notes.

_____

_____

_____

_____

_____

_____

Suggested Follow-Up Discussion

Your instructor may facilitate a discussion or presentation of your findings and discuss the different roles and responsibilities within the interprofessional team and the importance of interprofessional collaboration in providing high-quality care in the nursing home setting.

APPLICATION OF CONTENT IN THE CLINICAL AND/OR SIMULATION SETTING: Goals of Care Conversation in the Nursing Home

Simulation & Role-Play Activity

Your instructor will lead an in-class role-playing activity to explore possible responses to the scenario.

Objective

To help nursing students practice communication skills with older adults regarding goals of care, focusing on medical options and understanding the resident's wishes.

Description

Scenario: A quiet, private area in the nursing home, conducive to a sensitive conversation. Mr. Avery Jones is an 84-year-old resident with multiple medical conditions, including type 2 diabetes, chronic urinary incontinence, progressive dysphagia, and early-stage dementia. The social worker is meeting with him to discuss his goals of care and preferences for future medical decisions.

Roles:

1. Older adult resident (Mr. Avery Jones)
2. Social worker

Simulation Script

Social worker: *Greeting Mr. Jones warmly.* "Hi Mr. Jones, it's nice to see you today. I wanted to take some time to talk about your health and your wishes regarding your care. How are you feeling today?"

Mr. Jones: "I'm doing OK, just a bit tired. What do you want to talk about?"

Social worker: "I appreciate you sharing that. I want to understand more about your health and what's important to you when it comes to your care. Can we discuss your current medical conditions and how you feel about them?"

Mr. Jones: "Sure. I know I have diabetes, and the doctor said something about my swallowing getting worse. I sometimes feel frustrated because I can't do things I used to."

Social worker: "That's completely understandable. It can be challenging to adjust. Could you share how much you understand about your conditions right now and what they mean for your day-to-day life?"

Mr. Jones: "I know I have to watch what I eat for my diabetes, but sometimes I forget. And the swallowing... it just makes eating more complicated."

Social worker: "Thank you for sharing that. It's important to know how these conditions affect you. As we look ahead, I'd like to discuss your goals for care if your health were to worsen. What are some things that are important for you to consider if you find yourself in a more difficult situation?"

Mr. Jones: "I guess I want to make sure I'm not in pain. I wouldn't want any treatments that make me feel worse."

Social worker: "That's a very important consideration. Pain management is crucial. Are there any specific types of medical care or interventions you feel strongly about, either for or against?"

Mr. Jones: "I don't want to be hooked up to machines or anything. I'd rather be comfortable. But I also want to make sure I'm not a burden on my family."

Social worker: "Your comfort is a priority, and it's great that you're thinking about your family, too. Let's talk about your hopes and fears regarding healthcare. What worries you most when you think about your health and medical care?"

Mr. Jones: "I worry about forgetting things and not being able to speak up for myself. I don't want to feel alone in this."

Social worker: "Feeling supported is essential, and we can work together to ensure your wishes are known and respected. How do you feel about having a designated person, maybe a family member or friend, who can advocate for you if you can't speak for yourself?"

Mr. Jones: "That sounds good. My daughter would want to help. I just want to make sure she knows what I want."

Social worker: "That's a great plan. We can document your preferences and ensure your daughter is involved in these discussions. Is there anything else you'd like to share about your goals or concerns?"

Mr. Jones: "Just that I want to be comfortable and at peace. Thank you for listening."

Social worker: "Thank you for being open with me, Mr. Jones. This conversation is important, and I appreciate your trust. We'll keep working together to ensure your wishes are honored."

Debriefing Questions

Your instructor may use these questions as a group activity and class discussion, so consider the questions, record your responses below, and bring them to class.

For activities that will be done in class, as discussions or group activities, it is still beneficial to do some reflection before class to prepare.

1. How did you feel while role-playing your role?

   _____
   _____
   _____

2. What communication strategies were effective in facilitating the conversation?

   _____
   _____
   _____

3. Were there any challenges in discussing sensitive topics, and how were they addressed?

   _____
   _____
   _____

4. What did the social worker do well to make Mr. Jones feel comfortable sharing his thoughts and feelings?

5. How can this experience inform your future practice when discussing goals of care with older adults?

REFERENCE

Institute for Healthcare Improvement. (2020, July). *Age-friendly health systems: Guide to using the 4Ms in the care of older adults.* https://www.americangeriatrics.org/sites/default/files/inline-files/IHIAgeFriendlyHealthSystems_GuidetoUsing4MsCare.pdf09_

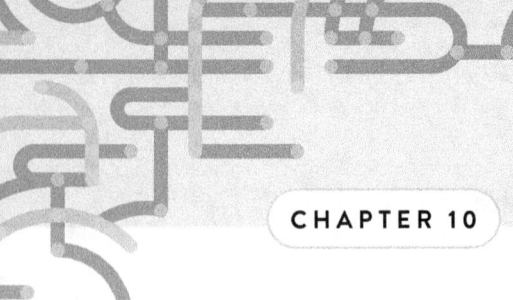

CHAPTER 10

REGULATORY CONTEXT

–Julie Britton, DNP, MSN, RN-BC, GCNS-BC, FGNLA; Jennifer Pyne; Kristin Mancini, MSNEd, RN, CRRN; Cathleen Soda, RN; Wendy Ness, MBA, NHA, QCP

BRIEF CHAPTER SUMMARY

Long-term care facilities in the United States operate under a complex web of federal and state regulations designed to ensure resident safety and quality care. Federal regulations, primarily through the Centers for Medicare & Medicaid Services (CMS), establish core standards for resident rights, quality of care, staffing, services, and facility management.

Nursing homes can effectively prepare for state surveys by adopting a proactive and comprehensive approach. This includes conducting regular internal audits and mock surveys to identify and address potential deficiencies beforehand. Facilities should ensure all staff members are trained in current regulations and the facility's policies and procedures, with a focus on resident rights and quality care practices. Fostering open communication and collaboration among staff, residents, and families creates a culture of transparency and encourages feedback for ongoing improvement. Staying abreast of any regulatory updates and incorporating them into daily practices ensures a state of continuous readiness for surveys.

> **CHAPTER LEARNING OUTCOMES**
> - Discuss how and why the OBRA '89/Nursing Home Reform Act and Final Rule was implemented
> - Define the purpose, types, and frequency of surveys conducted in long-term/post-acute care facilities
> - Describe the implications of survey results for a nursing home's Five Star Rating
> - Appreciate the relationship between regulatory requirements, quality care, and optimal resident outcomes

DISCUSSION QUESTIONS

Your instructor may use these questions as a group activity and class discussion, so consider the questions, record your responses below, and bring them to class.

For activities that will be done in class, as discussions or group activities, it is still beneficial to do some reflection before class to prepare.

1. Think about a recent interaction you had with a resident where you had to consider their rights and your responsibilities as a nurse. How did federal regulations (like those within the F-Tags) guide your actions in that situation?

   _____

   _____

   _____

   _____

2. Imagine you are a surveyor observing your own unit. Based on your current understanding of the survey process and common deficiencies, what areas do you think would receive the most scrutiny? What steps can you and the team take to proactively address those potential concerns?

   _____

   _____

   _____

   _____

NEXTGEN NCLEX STYLE QUESTIONS

1. A resident with dementia consistently refuses to take their medication. Which of the following actions is *most* important to ensure the facility remains compliant with federal regulations?

   a. Document the resident's refusal and inform the physician

   b. Crush the medication and mix it in the resident's food

   c. Restrain the resident and administer the medication

   d. Attempt to identify the reason for the refusal and explore alternative approaches

2. During a state survey, you observe a surveyor reviewing medication administration records (MARs). What are they *most* likely looking for to determine compliance with regulations?

   a. Neatness and legibility of the MARs

   b. Accuracy of the medication orders and documentation of administration

   c. Whether the MARs are electronic or on paper

   d. The number of PRN medications administered for each resident

3. A resident's family member complains that their loved one is not receiving adequate assistance with bathing. To which F-tag would this complaint *most* likely relate?

    a. F-Tag 684 Quality of Care

    b. F-Tag 677 Activities of Daily Living

    c. F-Tag 689 Accidents

    d. F-Tag 880 Infection Control

4. Which of the following is *not* a common area of focus during a state survey in a long-term care facility?

    a. Resident rights and dignity

    b. Facility financial records

    c. Infection prevention and control practices

    d. Nutritional status of residents

5. What is the *primary* purpose of the state survey process in long-term care facilities?

    a. To identify and penalize facilities for any deficiencies

    b. To ensure compliance with federal regulations and promote resident well-being

    c. To provide training opportunities for facility staff

    d. To gather data for research purposes

CASE STUDY: Dining Observation in a Nursing Home

Background

The regulation F550 Resident Rights states: "The facility must treat each resident with respect and dignity and care for each resident in a manner and in an environment that promotes maintenance or enhancement of his or her quality of life, recognizing each resident's individuality. The facility must protect and promote the rights of the resident" (CMS, 2024, §483.10(a)(1). The document that outlines F550 Resident Rights is the Centers for Medicare and Medicaid Services (CMS) State Operations Manual. F550, also known as "Resident Rights/Exercise of Rights," is a key part of the regulations governing long-term care facilities. This document ensures that residents in these facilities have the right to exercise their rights without interference, coercion, discrimination, or reprisal. It also outlines the rights of justice-involved individuals residing in these facilities, according to the CMS.

Scenario

Surveyors from the Centers for Medicare & Medicaid Services are conducting a routine inspection of a long-term care facility. During their visit, they observe meal service in the dining room, focusing on various aspects of the dining experience.

During the dining room meal, the surveyors observe two staff members assisting during the dining experience. When the trays arrive in the dining room, the staff start to pass the trays to different tables. The surveyors also observe the staff member using her bare hands to butter the resident's bread and then standing to provide feeding assistance to a resident. At the end of the meal, multiple residents are observed with clothes soiled with food and dried food on their hands.

Action

The observed actions of the staff indicate violations of infection control protocols and a lack of attention to resident dignity and cleanliness.

Interventions

- Educate staff on proper hand hygiene and food handling procedures
- Reinforce the importance of resident dignity and cleanliness during mealtimes
- Implement a system to ensure residents receive adequate assistance with eating and personal hygiene during and after meals
- Implement ongoing monitoring and auditing of mealtime practices
- Educate staff to use gloves or other appropriate utensils for food handling

Conclusion

The observations made during the survey suggest a need for improvement in the facility's dining services, particularly regarding infection control and resident dignity.

Questions

Your instructor may use these questions as a group activity and class discussion, so consider the questions, record your responses below, and bring them to class.

For activities that will be done in class, as discussions or group activities, it is still beneficial to do some reflection before class to prepare.

1. How might the observed practices impact resident dignity and quality of life?

_____

_____

_____

_____

2. What are the key components of proper hand hygiene and food handling in a long-term care setting?

3. What strategies can be implemented to improve the overall dining experience for residents?

4. How can the facility ensure ongoing compliance with infection control and resident regulations?

Reference

Centers for Medicare & Medicaid Services. (2024, August 8). *State operations manual Appendix PP: Guidance to surveyors for long term care facilities.* https://www.cms.gov/medicare/provider-enrollment-and-certification/guidanceforlawsandregulations/downloads/appendix-pp-state-operations-manual.pdf

IN-CLASS ACTIVITIES OR ASSIGNMENTS

Your instructor may assign these as in-class activities or as reflection activities done outside of class. For activities that will be done in class, as discussions or group activities, it is still beneficial to do some reflection before class to prepare.

Group Activity: Exploring Nursing Home Survey Types

Objective

To help nursing students understand the different types of surveys nursing homes encounter, their purpose, and the impact of each type of survey on care facilities.

Activity Overview

In this activity, nursing students will work in small groups to review real-life case scenarios and determine which type of survey applies to each situation. Students will categorize the surveys, discuss their purpose and focus areas, and then share their findings with the class.

Materials needed: A case study scenario handout for each group

Assignment Instructions

1. Your instructor will begin with a brief discussion on the importance of understanding the various nursing home survey types.

2. Your instructor will divide learners into small groups. Each group will receive a case scenario handout and will discuss and identify which survey type is most appropriate for each scenario. Each case scenario includes a brief description of a situation that a nursing home staff might encounter.

   Each group will:

   - Discuss each scenario and decide which type of survey applies
   - Identify the key elements of the scenario that led to their decision
   - Consider what the main focus of the survey would be in that case (e.g., resident rights, safety, care procedures)

3. Group presentation:

   After the group discussion, each group presents their findings to the class. For each scenario, the group should:

   - Share which survey type they selected
   - Explain why they chose that survey type, citing key facts from the scenario
   - Discuss any areas of concern they believe would be the focus of the survey (e.g., infection control, safety standards, staffing, etc.)

Discussion Questions

Your instructor may facilitate an in-class discussion or assign the following questions as discussion board topics. Use the space provided to record your notes.

1. How do the different survey types compare?

2. How might survey findings impact facility operations, care quality, and regulatory compliance?

3. What role do surveys have in improving patient care and ensuring safety in long-term care settings?

4. How do different survey types affect nursing staff and leadership?

5. Why are some facilities more likely to be subjected to special focus facility surveys?

_____

_____

_____

_____

6. How can a nursing home prepare for different types of surveys?

_____

_____

_____

_____

Case Study Scenario Handouts

Scenario 1: Infection Control Complaint

A family member calls to report that their loved one was not isolated during a respiratory outbreak, and they were exposed to other residents who tested positive for COVID-19. An investigation is initiated.

Survey type: Complaint survey

Focus: Infection control procedures and staff adherence to isolation protocols

Scenario 2: Fire Safety Violation

During a standard survey, surveyors find that the facility's fire alarm system has not been properly tested in over a year, violating the life safety code.

Survey type: Standard and life safety code survey

Focus: Compliance with life safety code standards, fire safety equipment, and emergency procedures

Scenario 3: Routine Survey

A nursing home undergoes a routine survey with no recent complaints or violations. The surveyor checks overall compliance with Medicare and Medicaid requirements.

Survey type: Standard survey

Focus: Broad assessment of regulatory compliance across all categories (resident rights, staffing, care procedures, etc.)

Scenario 4: Special Focus Facility

A nursing home has been found non-compliant in several recent surveys, and regulators have placed it on the special focus facilities list, which requires additional inspections.

Survey type: Special focus facility survey

Focus: Intensive scrutiny on areas where the facility has been repeatedly non-compliant (e.g., staffing, care quality, safety)

Conclusion

It is important that nurses understand the importance of being prepared for surveys and understanding how various survey types are designed to address different aspects of care and safety. They should also think critically about how they can contribute to ensuring compliance and improving quality of care in long-term care settings.

Brain Drain Activity: Daily Nursing Activities for a Safe and Compliant Environment

Objective

To help nursing students identify and understand the key daily and regular activities nurses must perform to ensure a safe, compliant environment for residents in long-term care settings.

Activity Overview

This is a "Brain Drain" style activity where nursing students will work individually or in small groups to brainstorm and list all the daily or regular activities they believe are essential to maintain a safe, compliant environment for residents in nursing homes. The activity encourages active recall and stimulates thinking about everyday practices and safety protocols.

Materials needed:
- Whiteboard or flip chart
- Markers
- Timer or clock
- Sticky notes (optional)
- Handouts or worksheets with prompt questions (optional)

Assignment Instructions

1. **Introduction:** Your instructor will begin with a brief discussion on the importance of being able to identify and discuss the daily or regular tasks that nurses must complete to ensure compliance with regulations, provide safe care, and protect the well-being of residents. A compliant environment involves adhering to regulatory standards, resident rights, safety protocols, infection control, documentation, and effective communication.

2. **Group activity:** Students will be divided by the instructor into small groups or asked as individuals to take a few minutes to think about and list as many activities as possible in response to the question, "What activities must a nurse do regularly to ensure safety, compliance, and quality care in a nursing home?"

3. **Sharing and discussion:** After the brainstorming session, the instructor may invite students to share their answers with their groups, present their top three to five activities, and write their responses on a whiteboard or flip chart. Alternatively, your instructor may ask each group to share their results with the class.

Discussion Questions

After the group presentations, your instructor may use these questions as a group activity and class discussion, so consider the questions, record your responses below, and bring them to class.

For activities that will be done in class, as discussions or group activities, it is still beneficial to do some reflection before class to prepare.

1. Why is this activity important for compliance and safety?

   _____

   _____

   _____

   _____

2. How does it contribute to resident well-being?

   _____

   _____

   _____

   _____

3. What specific regulations or standards does this activity address?

4. How does proper documentation contribute to regulatory compliance and resident care?

5. Why is infection control a critical daily task in nursing homes?

6. How does effective communication with residents, families, and staff contribute to a safe environment?

7. What are the most common activities that appeared on everyone's list?

8. Are there any activities that you initially overlooked (e.g., environmental safety checks, ensuring residents' rights, etc.)?

9. How do these daily tasks connect to broader concepts like quality of care, risk management, and patient safety?

Extension/Follow-Up Assignments & Activities

Your instructor may assign additional readings or case studies to explore these concepts further or assign one or both of the following:

- Learners write a brief reflection on how they would prioritize and organize these activities during a typical nursing shift.
- The instructor or the learners create role-play scenarios where nursing students practice the application of these activities in specific situations, such as managing an infection control outbreak or responding to a resident safety issue.

IN-CLASS ACTIVITIES OR ASSIGNMENTS FOR LEARNERS ALREADY FAMILIAR WITH NURSING HOME SETTINGS

Problem-Based Learning Activity: 2567 Scope and Severity

This in-class group activity is designed to apply methodology for assigning Scope and Severity using a sample CMS 2567 which includes deficiencies for F550 (Resident Rights), F580 (Notification of Changes), and F585 (Grievances).

Nursing homes must comply with federal Medicare and Medicaid requirements to continue receiving program payments. CMS and state agencies conduct regular surveys to identify deficiencies, which are assessed based on their scope and severity. This can range from minor issues to immediate threats to resident health or safety. When noncompliance is found, enforcement may include monetary fines or denial of payments. Facilities must return to compliance and those that fail to return within three months face payment denial for new admissions, and those that remain noncompliant after six months may be terminated from Medicare and Medicaid.

The CMS-2567 form, issued by the Centers for Medicare & Medicaid Services (CMS), documents deficiencies found during health care facility surveys and outlines the facility's Plan of Correction. It is used by state survey agencies, accrediting organizations, and CMS regional offices to record compliance issues based on Medicare, Medicaid, or CLIA standards. The form serves as both a notification to facilities of deficiencies and a place for them to propose corrective actions. It is essential for regulatory compliance and maintaining facility standards. Redacted versions have been made publicly available for certain health care facilities. See Figure 10.1 for an example (full copy here: https://www.cms.gov/medicare/cms-forms/cms-forms/cms-forms-items/cms008860).

In nursing home care, F550 (Resident Rights) ensures that all residents are treated with dignity, respect, and freedom from abuse or neglect, safeguarding their autonomy and quality of life. F580 (Notification of Changes) requires the facility to promptly inform residents, their doctors, and families about significant changes in a resident's condition, treatment, or room assignment. F585 (Grievances) guarantees that residents can voice complaints or concerns without fear of retaliation, and mandates that the facility investigates and resolves grievances promptly.

Activity Overview

Materials needed:

- CMS 2567 (Link to web-based form: https://www.cms.gov/medicare/cms-forms/cms-forms/cms-forms-items/cms008860)
- Scope and Severity Matrix examples can be found online and also in Table 10.1
- CMS downloads can be found here: https://www.cms.gov/Medicare/Provider-Enrollment-and-Certification/CertificationandComplianc/Downloads/SFFSCORINGMETHODOLOGY.pdf

TABLE 10.1 Assessment Factors Used to Determine the Seriousness of Deficiencies Matrix

	ISOLATED	PATTERN	WIDESPREAD
Immediate jeopardy to resident health or safety	**J** PoC Required	**K** PoC Required	**L** PoC Required
Actual harm that is not immediate	**G** PoC Required	**H** PoC Required	**I** PoC Required
No actual harm with potential for more than minimal harm that is not immediate jeopardy	**D** PoC Required	**E** PoC Required	**F** PoC Required
No actual harm with potential for minimal harm	**A** **No** PoC Required No remedies Commitment to Correct Not on CMS-2567	**B** PoC Required	**C** PoC Required

Substandard quality of care means one or more deficiencies related to participation requirements under §483.10 "Resident rights", paragraphs (a)(1) through (a)(2), (b)(1) through (b)(2), (e) (except for (e)(2), (e)(7), and (e)(8)), (f)(1) through (f)(3), (f)(5) through (f)(8), and (i) of this chapter; §483.12 of this chapter "Freedom from abuse, neglect, and exploitation"; §483.24 of this chapter "Quality of life"; §483.25 of this chapter "Quality of care"; §483.40 "Behavioral health services", paragraphs (b) and (d) of this chapter; §483.45 "Pharmacy services", paragraphs (d), (e), and (f) of this chapter; §483.70 "Administration", paragraph (p) of this chapter, and §483.80 "Infection control", paragraph (d) of this chapter, which constitute either immediate jeopardy to resident health or safety; a pattern of or widespread actual harm that is not immediate jeopardy; or a widespread potential for more than minimal harm, but less than immediate jeopardy, with no actual harm.

Substantial compliance

The scope and severity of nursing home deficiencies are assigned a letter-based point rating using a grid system (often called the *Scope and Severity Matrix*), which combines the levels of scope (Isolated, Pattern, Widespread) and severity (Levels A–L):

Severity levels:

- Level 1 (A–C): No actual harm, potential for minimal harm
- Level 2 (D–F): No actual harm, but potential for more than minimal harm
- Level 3 (G–I): Actual harm that is not immediate jeopardy
- Level 4 (J–L): Immediate jeopardy to resident health or safety

DEPARTMENT OF HEALTH AND HUMAN SERVICES		CENTERS FOR MEDICARE & MEDICAID SERVICES OMB NO. 0938-0391	
STATEMENT OF DEFICIENCIES AND PLAN OF CORRECTION	(X1) PROVIDER/SUPPLIER/CLIA IDENTIFICATION NUMBER:	(X2) MULTIPLE CONSTRUCTION A. BUILDING _____ B. WING _____	(X3) DATE SURVEY COMPLETED C
NAME OF PROVIDER OR SUPPLIER		STREET ADDRESS, CITY, STATE, ZIP CODE	

(X4) ID PREFIX TAG	SUMMARY STATEMENT OF DEFICIENCIES (EACH DEFICIENCY MUST BE PRECEDED BY FULL REGULATORY OR LSC IDENTIFYING INFORMATION)	ID PREFIX TAG	PROVIDER'S PLAN OF CORRECTION (EACH CORRECTIVE ACTION SHOULD BE CROSS-REFERENCED TO THE APPROPRIATE DEFICIENCY)	(X5) COMPLETION DATE
F550 SS = H	§483.10(a) Resident Rights. The resident has a right to a dignified existence, self-determination, and communication with and access to persons and services inside and outside the facility, including those specified in this section. §483.10(a)(1) A facility must treat each resident with respect and dignity and care for each resident in a manner and in an environment that promotes maintenance or enhancement of his or her quality of life, recognizing each resident's individuality. The facility must protect and promote the rights of the residents. §483.10(a)(2) The facility must provide equal access to quality care regardless of diagnosis, severity of condition, or payment source. A facility must establish and maintain identical policies and practices regarding transfer, discharge, and the provision of services under the State plan for all residents regardless of payment source. §483.10(b) Exercise of Rights. The resident has the right to exercise his or her rights as a resident of the facility and as a citizen or resident of the United States. §483.10(b)(1) The facility must ensure that the resident can exercise his or her rights without interference, coercion, discrimination, or reprisal from the facility.			

DEPARTMENT OF HEALTH AND HUMAN SERVICES
CENTERS FOR MEDICARE & MEDICAID SERVICES OMB NO. 0938-0391

STATEMENT OF DEFICIENCIES AND PLAN OF CORRECTION	(X1) PROVIDER/SUPPLIER/CLIA IDENTIFICATION NUMBER:	(X2) MULTIPLE CONSTRUCTION A. BUILDING _____ B. WING _____	(X3) DATE SURVEY COMPLETED C 02/23/2022
NAME OF PROVIDER OR SUPPLIER		STREET ADDRESS, CITY, STATE, ZIP CODE	

(X4) ID PREFIX TAG	SUMMARY STATEMENT OF DEFICIENCIES (EACH DEFICIENCY MUST BE PRECEDED BY FULL REGULATORY OR LSC IDENTIFYING INFORMATION)	ID PREFIX TAG	PROVIDER'S PLAN OF CORRECTION (EACH CORRECTIVE ACTION SHOULD BE CROSS-REFERENCED TO THE APPROPRIATE DEFICIENCY)	(X5) COMPLETION DATE
F550	Continued from page 1 §483.10(b)(2) The resident has the right to be free of interference, coercion, discrimination, and reprisal from the facility in exercising his or her rights and to be supported by the facility in the exercise of his or her rights as required under this subpart. This REQUIREMENT is not met as evidenced by: Based on observations, record review, cell phone video footage, resident and staff interview the facility failed to treat a resident in a dignified manner when a medication aide spoke rudely to the resident when he requested his medication (Resident #4), failed to treat residents in a dignified manner by not providing incontinence care when requested and double and triple briefing the residents (Resident 3, Resident #5, Resident #9, Resident #10, and Resident #11) for 6 of 9 residents reviewed. The residents stated that waiting on incontinence care and wearing multiple briefs made them feel bad, low and like less of a man, demeaning, embarrassed and degraded. The findings included: 1. Resident #4 was admitted to the facility on 10/26/21. Review of the admission Minimum Data Set (MDS) dated 10/28/21 revealed that Resident #4 was cognitively intact and was independent with activities of daily living. Resident #4 was interviewed on 02/02/22 at 12:19 PM. Resident #4 stated that he had been at the facility since October 2021 and "nighttime in the facility were the worst." He stated that the staff were rude and yelled and cussed him a lot. He stated that he was paralyzed in a car accident in 2004 and had very bad back spasms which were exacerbated when he did not get his medication. He explained that at home he had			

FIGURE 10.1 CMS-2567 form.

Scope levels:

- Isolated: Affects one or few residents (A, D, G, J)
- Pattern: Affects more than a few residents (B, E, H, K)
- Widespread: Affects many or all residents (C, F, I, L)

Each combination (e.g., "G" for actual harm, isolated) corresponds to a specific enforcement weight. Ratings in the J–L range (immediate jeopardy) trigger the most severe enforcement actions, including immediate penalties or termination from Medicare/Medicaid (see Table 10.1).

Scope and Severity Scenario

Summary of Deficient Practice reported on CMS 2567:

The facility failed to ensure dignity and respect for six of nine sampled residents (Residents #3, #4, #5, #9, #10, and #11) because:

1. Resident #4 was not treated respectfully by medication aide (MA) #1, who spoke rudely, delayed medication administration, and used profanity when the resident requested medications for severe back spasms. A cell phone video confirmed MA #1's dismissive and inappropriate response. Although the incident was reported to administration and nursing leadership, there was no evidence of appropriate follow-up or resolution.

2. Residents #3, #5, #9, #10, and #11 experienced significant delays in incontinence care, ranging from 1.5 to 3.5 hours. Residents described feelings of shame, embarrassment, and being degraded from waiting in soiled briefs. Several residents were routinely dressed in two or even three briefs at once as a coping strategy due to infrequent care. One resident (#5) reported wearing three briefs because "staff don't come back for hours." Surveyor observation and staff interviews confirmed this.

3. Resident #11's call light was reportedly on for over 3 hours (from 7:30 p.m. to after 11:00 p.m.) without staff response, leading the resident's family to call the police for a wellness check. The resident remained wet throughout this time and described the incident as "demeaning."

4. Staff interviews: Several nurse aides admitted to using double/triple briefing to compensate for lack of timely care. Staff cited inadequate staffing levels, being unable to meet 2-hour check-and-change expectations, and delays caused by conflicting meal service responsibilities. One aide confirmed she only changed a resident once during her entire shift due to workload.

5. Leadership response: The DON and Administrator acknowledged care delays and agreed that wearing multiple briefs and leaving residents in soiled conditions were unacceptable. However, staffing constraints and poor communication contributed to ongoing dignity-related care issues. The DON stated that increasing the frequency of incontinence checks was necessary, and the Administrator indicated plans to contract more reliable agency staff.

Assignment Instructions

Your instructor will guide the group activities, including providing copies of the Sample 2567 and a Scope and Severity Matrix table to assign the appropriate scope and severity to each of the FTag deficiencies.

When the allotted time is up, the instructor will review the answers for each citation. Students will self-grade their answers.

Debriefing

1. What did you find surprising about this activity?

   _____

   _____

   _____

   _____

2. What can you take away for next time you need to review a CMS 2567?

   _____

   _____

   _____

   _____

Plan of Correction Add-on Learning Activity

F550 – SS=H—Resident Rights: Dignity and Respect

Following the models reviewed in the previous activity and discussion, your instructor may direct learners to create a Plan of Correction similar to the sample below.

Plan of Correction Example

Tag #: F550
Regulation: §483.10(a)-(b)
Completion Date: [Insert Date – typically 30–45 days from citation date]
Facility Name: [Insert Facility Name]
Survey Date: [Insert Survey Date]

1. Corrective action for affected residents:
   - Resident #4:
     - Immediately evaluated by the Social Services Director and DON.
     - Counseling offered to address emotional distress related to the incident.
     - Medication aide (MA #1) was removed from direct care responsibilities pending investigation.
     - Education provided to staff regarding respectful communication and timely medication delivery.
   - Residents #3, #5, #9, #10, and #11:
     - All received full skin assessments to evaluate for breakdown due to prolonged soiling.
     - Incontinence care frequency increased to every two hours and as needed.
     - Call light systems were tested and confirmed operational; documentation of call response times began immediately.
     - Resident interviews conducted by social services to assess emotional impact and provide support.

2. Systemic measures to ensure future compliance:
   - Inservice education: All nursing staff (including aides and medication aides) are re-educated on:
     - Resident rights (dignity, respect, freedom from abuse and neglect)
     - Timely response to call lights and incontinence needs
     - Prohibition of multiple brief use except by resident choice with clinical justification
   - Staffing adjustments:
     - Staffing patterns are reviewed and adjusted to ensure adequate coverage during peak hours.
     - A new agency is contracted to provide supplemental staffing while permanent recruitment is underway.
   - Communication and reporting protocols:
     - Staff is reminded of the requirement to report all allegations of verbal abuse or neglect immediately to the Administrator or DON.
     - A daily Quality of Life Rounds sheet is implemented to proactively identify residents with unmet dignity needs.

3. Monitoring to ensure ongoing compliance:
    - Daily audits: Unit managers or charge nurses will conduct daily random audits of five residents per unit for:
        - Timeliness of incontinence care
        - Call light response (goal: <10-minute response)
        - Use of appropriate number of briefs
        - Staff interaction/communication tone
    - Weekly resident interviews: Social Services will interview five residents weekly for four weeks, then monthly x three months, asking:
        - Do you feel respected by staff?
        - Are your needs met in a timely manner?
    - QA Committee oversight:
        - Findings will be reviewed weekly in the Quality Assurance and Performance Improvement (QAPI) committee.
        - Adjustments will be made based on audit results or any new grievances.
4. Responsible party: The DON is responsible for ensuring the implementation and maintenance of this Plan of Correction.

APPLICATION OF CONTENT IN THE CLINICAL AND/OR SIMULATION SETTING: Five Scenarios for Identifying and Correcting Deficiencies in Care Provided in the Nursing Home

Your instructor will lead an in-class role-playing activity to explore possible responses to one or more of the following scenarios.

Objectives

- These scenarios provide valuable opportunities for staff education, training and collaboration.
- They allow for the identification of potential survey deficiencies and prompt corrective action.
- They reinforce the importance of adhering to policies and procedures.
- They promote a culture of continuous quality improvement in the facility.

Description

These scenarios can be used as in-class or clinical discussion prompts. For example, if learners experience a scenario in the clinical setting like one of the scenarios below, they could be used in post-clinical debriefing. They can also be used as the base for clinical simulation scenarios. Brief instructions are provided below on how these might be expanded for use as simulations.

Scenario One: Walking Rounds to Identify Areas of Deficient Practice

Scenario: During a mock survey, the team—including a nurse, an administrator, and a social worker—conduct walking rounds. In a resident's room, they find an overflowing wastebasket, a call light out of reach, prescription medication on a nightstand, and a spill on the floor that hasn't been cleaned.

Application: This scenario highlights deficiencies in housekeeping, resident safety (call light access), and storage of medication and infection control (unattended spill). It provides an opportunity to educate staff on these areas and reinforce the importance of proactive rounds to identify and address potential hazards.

Materials: Mock survey forms or observation checklists

Roles: Nurse, administrator, and social worker

Debriefing Questions

Your instructor may use these questions as a group activity and class discussion, so consider the questions, record your responses below, and bring them to class.

For activities that will be done in class, as discussions or group activities, it is still beneficial to do some reflection before class to prepare.

1. What hazards or deficiencies did you observe?

   _____

   _____

   _____

2. What are the risks to resident safety in this scenario?

   _____

   _____

   _____

3. What immediate actions should be taken?

4. How can proactive rounding improve care quality?

Scenario Two: Medication Administration Observations

Scenario: A simulated medication pass is observed. The nurse is seen administering medication without verifying the resident's identity and then failing to document the medication given.

Application: This simulation reveals critical errors in medication administration. It allows for immediate feedback to the nurse, emphasizing the "five rights" of medication administration and the importance of accurate documentation. It also prompts a review of medication administration policies and procedures.

Materials: Handout of resident chart with medication orders; checklist for observers to document errors

Roles: Nurse, resident

Debriefing Questions

Your instructor may use these questions as a group activity and class discussion, so consider the questions, record your responses below, and bring them to class.

For activities that will be done in class, as discussions or group activities, it is still beneficial to do some reflection before class to prepare.

1. What were the errors made during the medication pass?

2. Which of the "five rights" were violated?

3. Why is documentation immediately after administration critical?

4. What are strategies to prevent medication errors?

Scenario Three: Wound Care Observations

Scenario: A wound care nurse is observed performing a dressing change on a simulated wound. The nurse doesn't perform proper hand hygiene before and after the procedure, and the used, heavily soiled dressings are disposed of in the trash receptacle and left in the resident's room.

Application: This simulation demonstrates non-compliance with infection control protocols. It provides a chance to re-educate the nurse on proper hand hygiene techniques and the correct disposal of contaminated materials. It also highlights the need for ongoing monitoring of wound care practices.

Materials: Mannequin or simulation model with a mock wound, wound care supplies (gloves, gauze, hand sanitizer, etc.)

Roles: Nurse

Debriefing Questions

Your instructor may use these questions as a group activity and class discussion, so consider the questions, record your responses below, and bring them to class.

For activities that will be done in class, as discussions or group activities, it is still beneficial to do some reflection before class to prepare.

1. What infection control breaches occurred?

   _____

   _____

   _____

2. Why is proper disposal of contaminated materials critical?

   _____

   _____

   _____

3. What policies address wound care hygiene?

   _____

   _____

   _____

4. What could have been done differently in this scenario?

   _____

   _____

   _____

Scenario Four: Proper Feeding of Residents in a Dining Room Setting

Scenario: Observers in the dining room notice a resident struggling to eat their meal due to limited dexterity. A staff member places the food tray in front of the resident and leaves without offering assistance or alerting a nurse.

Application: This scenario illustrates a failure to provide adequate assistance with meals. It prompts a discussion about the importance of assessing residents' needs and providing appropriate support, such as adaptive utensils, assistance with cutting food, or offering alternative food choices.

Materials: Dining area set, hand splint or gloves

Roles: Dining staff member, resident with limited mobility, residents dining (observers)

Debriefing Questions

Your instructor may use these questions as a group activity and class discussion, so consider the questions, record your responses below, and bring them to class.

For activities that will be done in class, as discussions or group activities, it is still beneficial to do some reflection before class to prepare.

1. What was inappropriate about the staff's response?

2. What should staff do when a resident shows difficulty eating?

3. How does mealtime support impact nutrition and dignity?

4. What training is needed for dining staff?

Scenario Five: Restorative Nursing Care

Scenario: A resident who recently experienced a stroke is observed during a restorative nursing session. The certified nursing assistant (CNA) is assisting the resident with range-of-motion exercises but is performing passive range-of-motion rather than assisting the patient with active range-of-motion, causing the resident discomfort.

Application: This simulation identifies a need for further training on proper restorative nursing techniques. It allows for immediate correction of the CNA's technique and emphasizes the importance of resident comfort and safety during these activities. It also highlights the need for ongoing competency assessments for staff providing restorative care.

Materials needed: Range-of-motion tools

Roles: CNA, resident

Debriefing Questions

Your instructor may use these questions as a group activity and class discussion, so consider the questions, record your responses below, and bring them to class.

For activities that will be done in class, as discussions or group activities, it is still beneficial to do some reflection before class to prepare.

1. What technique errors were observed?

2. Why is it important to differentiate passive vs. active ROM?

3. What risks come from improper ROM exercises?

4. How can staff ensure safety during restorative care?

REFERENCE

Centers for Medicare & Medicaid Services. (2024, Aug. 8). *State operations manual Appendix PP: Guidance to surveyors for long term care facilities.* https://www.cms.gov/medicare/provider-enrollment-and-certification/guidanceforlawsandregulations/downloads/appendix-pp-state-operations-manual.pdf

CHAPTER 11

FINANCING SENIOR LIVING SERVICES AND LONG-TERM CARE

–Nancy D. Zionts, MBA; Sophie A. Campbell, MSN, RN, CRRN, RAC-CT, CNDLTC; Brian Stever, BSN, RN, RAC-CT

BRIEF CHAPTER SUMMARY

Understanding the financing of long-term care (LTC) is essential for nursing staff, as their clinical practices and documentation play a pivotal role in facility reimbursement and the overall funding of care. Nurses are often the frontline professionals whose assessments, notes, and interventions directly influence the financial health of LTC facilities. This knowledge is not only relevant for day-to-day responsibilities but is also crucial for career advancement, particularly for those aiming to transition into administrative or leadership roles. Accurate documentation, driven by sound clinical judgment and high-quality care, ensures that facilities receive appropriate compensation and reinforces the value of the nursing profession within the broader healthcare system.

LTC financing is complex, involving various payors and reimbursement arrangements. Facilities must navigate structures like fee-for-service models, global payments, and incentive-based programs. Primary sources of reimbursement include private pay, where residents or their families pay directly; Medicare, which funds skilled nursing and specific services; Medicare Advantage Plans, which offer similar coverage with additional requirements; and Medicaid, a state-managed program covering long-term residents' essential needs. Facilities are reimbursed for a broad spectrum of services, such as room and board, meals, medical supplies, medications, social services, rehabilitation therapies, and specific treatments.

A key aspect of this process is understanding the source of payment upon a resident's admission, which directly affects reimbursement accuracy and timeliness. Since October 1, 2019, nursing home payment structures have evolved under the Patient-Driven Payment Model (PDPM), replacing traditional fee-for-service and per diem Prospective Payment Systems (PPS). PDPM emphasizes resident needs and complexity over volume of services, with reimbursement rates determined by components such as medical diagnoses, therapy requirements, and functional abilities. This model includes six categories—Physical Therapy, Occupational Therapy, Speech-Language Pathology, Nursing, Non-therapy ancillary, and Non-Case Mix—organized into roughly 28,000 Case Mix Groupers used for payment classification.

The cornerstone of accurate PDPM reimbursement is the Minimum Data Set (MDS) 3.0, a standardized assessment tool used in skilled nursing facilities (SNFs). MDS documentation must reflect the clinical reality of the resident, integrating medical history, current conditions, and care needs. Proper use of electronic health records, daily notes, and comprehensive weekly summaries ensures that documentation supports the necessity for skilled nursing services and therapy intensity, especially when residents are covered under Medicare Part A. For coverage, residents must meet criteria such as having a qualifying hospital stay, needing daily skilled care confirmed by a physician, and receiving care in a Medicare-certified facility. Skilled services may include stroke recovery, Parkinson's disease management, wound care, and rehabilitation for acute conditions.

Ultimately, good documentation practices are not just a regulatory requirement—they are vital to ensuring proper reimbursement and sustaining the financial health of LTC organizations. By prioritizing clinical excellence, precise documentation, and an understanding of the reimbursement landscape, nursing staff can significantly contribute to both patient outcomes and the operational success of their facilities.

CHAPTER LEARNING OUTCOMES
- Differentiate between qualifications and payment for short-term post-acute care versus long-term care in nursing homes
- Appreciate the nurse's role in timely and accurate documentation in the health record to support nursing home reimbursement
- Describe the structure and contribution of the Minimum Data Set (MDS) in payment to nursing homes for care delivered
- Delineate the differences between nonprofit and for-profit nursing homes

DISCUSSION QUESTIONS

Your instructor may use these questions as a group activity and class discussion, so consider the questions, record your responses below, and bring them to class.

For activities that will be done in class, as discussions or group activities, it is still beneficial to do some reflection before class to prepare.

1. Why is it important for each nurse to know something about financial management and reimbursement for the nursing home?

   _____
   _____
   _____
   _____

2. Can nurses have an impact on financial management in the nursing home?

3. Should the reimbursement type for a resident influence the type/level of care you provide as a nurse?

4. How would you react if you were asked as a nurse to use different medical supplies on a resident based on their payor source to the nursing home?

5. How would you react if you were told that medication was denied a resident because of the cost and the payor refused to cover it while the resident was in the nursing home?

6. How would you respond if a resident was told that they either had to discharge from their short stay skilled nursing home stay or pay privately because the payor source would no longer cover the care and services being provided?

_____

_____

_____

_____

7. Where do you see the intersection of medical record documentation and reimbursement? Does it make sense for reimbursement to rely on documentation?

_____

_____

_____

_____

NEXTGEN NCLEX STYLE QUESTIONS

1. A nursing home resident is eligible for Medicare coverage for SNF services. Which condition must be met for the resident to qualify for this benefit?

    a. The resident must require custodial care.

    b. The resident must have had a qualifying hospital stay of at least three days.

    c. The resident must be under 65 years of age.

    d. The resident must have a private insurance plan.

2. A nursing home administrator is reviewing reimbursement methods for services provided to residents. Which payment model is most used for long-term care services in nursing homes?

    a. Per diem rate

    b. Fee-for-service

    c. Bundled payments

    d. Capitation

3. A nurse is assessing a new resident's financial situation to help determine eligibility for Medicaid. Which factor is most critical in this assessment?

    a. The resident's prior employment history

    b. The resident's monthly income and assets

    c. The resident's age and health status

    d. The resident's family support system

4. A nursing home nurse is educating staff about the implications of the Patient-Driven Payment Model (PDPM) on resident care. What is a key aspect of PDPM that nursing staff should understand?

    a. It eliminates the need for documentation.

    b. It focuses on the resident's diagnosis and care needs rather than volume of services.

    c. It guarantees full payment regardless of services provided.

    d. It requires daily assessments for reimbursement.

5. A nursing home resident's family is concerned about the costs of care. What should the nurse advise them regarding the potential for financial assistance?

    a. Financial assistance is not available for nursing home care.

    b. Only private insurance can help cover costs.

    c. They should explore Medicaid options and veteran benefits.

    d. Assistance is guaranteed for all residents regardless of income.

CASE STUDY: The Benefits of Accurate Documentation in Skilled Nursing Facilities for the Minimum Data Set Process

Background

Sunrise Skilled Nursing Facility (SSNF) is a reputable long-term care facility that accommodates Medicare A residents, providing skilled nursing and rehabilitation services. Recognizing the critical importance of accurate documentation, SSNF has recently implemented a new initiative aimed at enhancing the accuracy of its documentation processes, specifically focusing on the MDS assessments. This initiative is designed to improve the quality of care, ensure regulatory compliance, and enhance financial outcomes for Medicare A residents.

Patient Profile

Name: Mrs. Jane Doe

Age: 78

Diagnosis: Post-operative hip replacement, diabetes, hypertension

Admission date: March 1, 2024

Functional status: Requires assistance with activities of daily living (ADLs), including bathing, dressing, and ambulation

Scenario

Upon admission, Mrs. Jane Doe underwent her initial MDS assessment, which provided a comprehensive overview of her medical history, functional abilities, and the treatments and interventions required for her recovery. However, prior to the implementation of the accurate documentation initiative, SSNF faced several significant challenges:

- Incomplete records: Essential information regarding Jane's prior functional status and specific care needs was missing or inaccurately recorded, leading to potential gaps in her care plan.
- Inaccurate coding: Errors in coding could result in improper reimbursement rates and affect the facility's compliance with Medicare regulations.
- Delayed updates: Changes in Mrs. Doe's condition were not promptly documented, which hindered timely adjustments to her care plan, potentially impacting her recovery.

Implementation of Accurate Documentation

1. Comprehensive staff training sessions: SSNF conducted training sessions for all nursing and administrative staff focused on accurate documentation practices. These sessions included:
    - Detailed workshops on the MDS assessment process and its implications for resident care.
    - Case studies illustrating the consequences of poor documentation, including potential financial penalties and decreased quality of care.
    - Emphasis on detailed entries: Staff were trained to prioritize detailed and timely entries in resident records, reinforcing the significance of thorough documentation for regulatory compliance and optimal patient outcomes.

2. Technological upgrades: SSNF implemented a state-of-the-art advanced electronic health record system to streamline data entry and retrieval processes. Features included:
    - User-friendly interfaces for easy navigation and documentation.
    - Automated prompts to guide staff in completing necessary sections of the MDS assessment.

- Real-time data verification tools: The new system included tools for real-time data verification to ensure accuracy in documentation. These tools:
    - Alerted staff to inconsistencies or missing information as data was entered.
    - Provided instant feedback, allowing for immediate corrections and updates.

3. Impact of the initiative: Following the implementation of the accurate documentation initiative, SSNF observed several positive outcomes:
    - Improved quality of care: With accurate and timely documentation, Jane's care plan was more effectively tailored to her needs. Nurses were able to adjust her interventions based on real-time assessments, leading to improved functional outcomes.
    - Regulatory compliance: Accurate coding of diagnoses and treatment plans resulted in better compliance with Medicare regulations, minimizing the risk of audits and penalties.
    - Enhanced financial outcomes: Improved documentation led to appropriate reimbursement rates for services provided, supporting the facility's financial stability.

Questions

Your instructor may use these questions as a group activity and class discussion, so consider the questions, record your responses below, and bring them to class.

For activities that will be done in class, as discussions or group activities, it is still beneficial to do some reflection before class to prepare.

1. What are the potential consequences of inaccurate documentation for both residents and the facility?

   _____

   _____

   _____

2. How can the implementation of technology improve the documentation process in SNFs?

   _____

   _____

   _____

3. What strategies can nursing staff use to ensure that documentation remains accurate and up to date?

4. In what ways does accurate documentation impact interdisciplinary communication and collaboration?

5. How can facilities measure the success of initiatives aimed at improving documentation practices?

IN-CLASS ACTIVITIES OR ASSIGNMENTS

Your instructor may assign these as in-class activities or as reflection activities done outside of class.

For activities that will be done in class, as discussions or group activities, it is still beneficial to do some reflection before class to prepare.

Learning Activity: Care vs. Cost Scenario & Discussion

This assignment may be done in class as a group activity or role-play, discussion, or assigned as an individual project.

This scenario underscores the ongoing challenge healthcare professionals face when navigating between high-quality care and financial constraints. It is vital to advocate for the resident's health while also being mindful of the financial impact on both the resident and the healthcare facility. This situation reminds me of the importance of open communication among the care team and the need for a collaborative approach when addressing complex medical decisions. Ultimately, our goal should be to ensure that residents receive the best possible care while also considering their financial wellbeing and exploring all available options.

Scenario

You are the unit manager registered nurse. You receive an admission from the hospital and are reviewing the transfer sheet from the hospital. You write the orders to correlate with the transfer sheet from the hospital which matches what you saw in the medical record while the resident was still a patient in the hospital.

You type in the orders and send them to the attending physician for review and approval. The physician approves all orders on admission. The list of medications includes an antibiotic for the diagnosis of VRE. You are not familiar with the antibiotic and call the pharmacy to ask about it. The pharmacy tells you that the antibiotic is usually given when several other antibiotics have been ineffective.

The next call you receive is from the pharmacy to let you know the antibiotic is very expensive at greater than $2,000 per dose, and the resident is ordered the antibiotic twice daily. You contact the attending physician who requests that you contact the hospital and see what the referring physician wants to do. The hospital tells you that the referring physician cannot change the antibiotic. The resident has been admitted and is in your facility. The resident is paying for care privately and is not covered by a third party payor.

Discussion Question

Your instructor may facilitate an in-class discussion or assign the following question as a discussion board topic.

How do you manage this situation that may be a care vs. cost dilemma? How do you respond and what are your thoughts about this situation?

_____

_____

_____

_____

Learning Activity: Care vs. Loss of Reimbursement Scenario & Discussion

This assignment may be done in class as a group activity or role-play, discussion, or assigned as an individual project.

This scenario highlights a significant ethical dilemma in healthcare which is balancing quality patient care with the constraints of reimbursement policies. It is disheartening to see financial considerations taking precedence over patient safety and well-being. As healthcare providers, we must advocate for our residents and ensure that they receive the necessary support to transition safely to their next phase of care. It is vital to engage with payors and policymakers to emphasize the need for patient-centered policies that prioritize health outcomes over cost savings. Ultimately, the residents' safety and quality of life should guide our decisions.

Scenario

You are the unit manager RN, and you are sitting in a weekly meeting with the interdisciplinary team discussing the resident's discharge plan. You learn in the meeting that the payor that provides reimbursement to the facility for the resident's short-term stay care has stated that the resident has two days left in their stay, and then they will no longer be covered and either be discharged from the facility or remain in your care without reimbursement.

The rehabilitation therapists state that they are willing to discharge the resident based on the payor recommendation. You asked the therapists if they have completed education with the resident and/or spouse regarding functional mobility and self-care tasks at home and their response is no. You discuss with the interdisciplinary team that, from your observations of the resident and what you have reviewed in the medical record from nursing over the three shifts notes, the resident is unable to perform self-care tasks, requires assist of one for all self-care, and has fallen on the night shift when walking to the bathroom, which he will have to do at home.

The full interdisciplinary team stated that they have no choice based on the decision by the payor to stop reimbursement for care and services in two days. All team members were prepared to sign off on the discharge.

Discussion Questions

Your instructor may facilitate an in-class discussion or assign the following questions as discussion board topics.

For activities that will be done in class, as discussions or group activities, it is still beneficial to do some reflection before class to prepare.

1. How would you respond to this? What options do you have?

_____

_____

_____

_____

2. How would you discuss this with the resident and family?

3. What are your thoughts about this care vs. payment dilemma?

APPLICATION OF CONTENT IN THE CLINICAL AND/OR SIMULATION SETTING: Balancing Clinical Care and Reimbursement Realities in a Skilled Nursing Facility

The following activity has been developed to be used as part of the clinical experience or as a simulation. Alternatively, the activity can be done in-class as a group activity or role-play, discussion, or assigned as an individual project. The activity can be used as a whole or broken into smaller discussions or assignments as well.

Objectives

- Practice effective communication with residents and families
- Learn strategies for safe and appropriate discharges
- Understand the importance of accurate documentation for reimbursement purposes.
- Collaborate effectively with interdisciplinary teams to advocate for our residents and ensure their needs are met, even when faced with obstacles such as payor denials or discrepancies in medical records

Description

As healthcare professionals working in nursing homes, it is essential to navigate the complexities of patient care while also understanding the financial and administrative aspects of practice. In this clinical setting, nurses play a pivotal role not only in delivering quality care but also in advocating for residents' needs, particularly concerning discharge planning and reimbursement issues. The transition from an SNF back to the community or to a lower level of care can be challenging, and it is crucial for nurses to ensure that residents are adequately prepared and supported throughout this process.

During pre- and post-conference discussions, we will explore various scenarios that may arise in daily practice. These discussions will center around key topics such as effective communication with residents and families, strategies for safe and appropriate discharges, and the importance of accurate documentation for reimbursement purposes. We will also address how to collaborate effectively with interdisciplinary teams to advocate for residents and ensure their needs are met, even when faced with obstacles such as payor denials or discrepancies in medical records.

By engaging in these discussions, we aim to foster a deeper understanding of the interplay between clinical care and the business of healthcare. This will enhance our ability to provide holistic, patient-centered care while also meeting regulatory requirements and securing necessary resources for residents. We encourage you to reflect on your experiences, share insights, and consider how the principles discussed can be applied in your practice. Together, we can strengthen our skills in navigating the multifaceted landscape of nursing home care, ensuring that residents receive the best possible outcomes.

Pre-Simulation Preparation

Pre-Readings/Resources

These readings can help you think more about payment structures for SNF and nursing home settings. They can help you engage in the pre and post simulation or clinical discussion questions provided here or your instructor may use them as resources in a different assignment structure.

1. Overview of Medicare Part A: https://www.medicare.gov/coverage/skilled-nursing-facility-care
2. PDMP in SNF: https://www.cms.gov/medicare/payment/prospective-payment-systems/skilled-nursing-facility-snf/patient-driven-model
3. Guide to Discharge Planning Best Practices: https://www.medicare.gov/coverage/nursing-home-care
4. Review of Minimum Data Set (MDS) and Reimbursement: https://www.cms.gov/medicare/payment/prospective-payment-systems/skilled-nursing-facility-snf/patient-driven-model
5. Additional Information: https://www.medicare.gov/providers-services/original-medicare/skilled-nursing

Reflection Questions for Pre-Simulation or Pre-Clinical Conference Settings

1. Have you participated in a resident discharge or care transition before? What challenges did you notice?

2. How does the documentation you complete affect reimbursement?

3. What is the nurse's role in advocating for a resident whose discharge might be financially or clinically inappropriate?

Simulation Scenario

Patient name: Mrs. Evelyn Thompson

Age: 84

Diagnosis: Stroke (left-sided weakness), hypertension, dementia (mild)

Admitted to the SNF 20 days ago for a stay covered under Medicare Part A

Situation summary and script:

Mrs. Thompson was admitted to the SNF after a three-day acute care stay following a stroke. She has received daily skilled PT, OT, and nursing services. Recently, the interdisciplinary team determined she may be ready for discharge back to her own home within three days. The care team, however, is facing two key issues:

1. Family concerns: Her daughter believes she is not ready to come home and has requested additional SNF days.

2. Payor constraints: Medicare will not cover additional days unless skilled services are justified. The latest MDS documentation does not clearly support continued skilled need.

You, as the nurse, are responsible for:

- Communicating with the family about the discharge plan and reimbursement limitations.

- Collaborating with the interdisciplinary team to review documentation for justification of continued stay (if clinically appropriate).

- Ensuring proper documentation for reimbursement or preparing for a safe transition to home.

Simulation setup:

Roles:

- Nurse (student/participant)
- Resident's daughter (played by facilitator or actor)
- Social worker (played by another student or facilitator)
- MDS coordinator (optional role)
- Charge nurse or unit manager

Props, as available:
- Sample chart with medical notes, therapy progress, and incomplete MDS
- Medicare coverage guidelines printout
- Discharge summary draft
- Nursing notes template

Role-Play Activity

Your instructor will lead an in-class role-playing activity to explore possible responses to the scenario.

Post-Simulation Debriefing Questions

Your instructor may use these questions as a group activity and class discussion, so consider the questions, record your responses below, and bring them to class.

For activities that will be done in class, as discussions or group activities, it is still beneficial to do some reflection before class to prepare.

1. How do you discuss discharge with a resident that is earlier than you expected based on what you know about the resident's functional mobility and self-care abilities?

   _____

   _____

   _____

   _____

2. How can the nurse assist the resident to be prepared for a safe and appropriate discharge?

   _____

   _____

   _____

   _____

3. How can the nurse ensure the resident and family understand the rationale for the payor stopping reimbursement when they don't think the resident is ready?

4. What should the nurse do when you review medical record documentation that is not accurate regarding the care and services provided to the resident?

5. How can the nurse assist the interdisciplinary team to understand when the resident is safe and appropriate for discharge based on functional mobility and self-care?

6. What can the nurse do when the payor will not cover the cost of medications for the resident because of cost, but the physician states the resident requires the medications and no other medication can be administered?

7. What can the nurse do when documentation is not completed for several days for a short-term skilled stay resident, and documentation supports the MDS assessment which supports reimbursement?

8. What can the nurse do when the MDS assessment in the medical record notes items coded that are not accurate to represent the care and services of the resident and does not correlate to the medial record documentation?

CHAPTER 12

IMPROVING QUALITY IN NURSING HOMES

–Melissa Batchelor, PhD, RN-BC, FNP-BC, FGSA, FAAN

BRIEF CHAPTER SUMMARY

In the United States, nursing homes serve as a crucial part of the long-term care system, providing both healthcare and residential services to older adults with complex medical needs. Despite regulations and efforts to enhance care, the industry continues to face challenges related to quality and safety, underscored by high-profile issues during the COVID-19 pandemic.

A primary focus of this chapter is the role of quality measures in evaluating and improving nursing home performance and their culture of safety. The Centers for Medicare & Medicaid Services (CMS) has established quality measures that assess various aspects of resident care, including clinical outcomes, safety, and patient satisfaction. These measures are publicly reported through tools like Medicare's Care Compare website, empowering consumers to make informed choices and holding facilities accountable. The chapter also describes the process for implementing quality improvement programs in nursing homes and explains the National Academies of Sciences, Engineering, and Medicine's (NASEM) conceptual model of quality in nursing homes. The standardization and transparency of these aggregated measures is one form of individual nursing home accountability, and the information is a starting point to help consumers make informed decisions about the quality and safety available in their local area (or nationally for distance-based caregivers). However, while this public service helps consumers make some decisions about how local nursing homes perform in comparison to state and national averages, the voices and experiences of quality of life by residents and families are not captured (e.g., factors like a homelike environment, food quality, and social engagement).

This chapter includes teaching and learning materials that combine external, publicly available data with site visits to capture the voice and lived experiences of families and residents. The resources and learning activities are intended to make this typically overwhelming information into an experience students can teach at the bedside and/or provide valuable educational resources to families needing to make this decision in the middle of a health crisis.

> **CHAPTER LEARNING OUTCOMES**
> - Explain the purpose of quality measure for nursing home care
> - Define the measures used to assess a facility's culture of safety
> - Describe the process for implementing QI programs in nursing homes
> - Explain the NASEM conceptual model of quality of care in nursing homes

DISCUSSION QUESTIONS

Your instructor may use these questions as a group activity and class discussion, so consider the questions, record your responses below, and bring them to class.

For activities that will be done in class, as discussions or group activities, it is still beneficial to do some reflection before class to prepare.

1. What role do quality measures play in improving the overall reputation and public perception of nursing homes?

   _____
   _____
   _____

2. How do short-stay and long-stay quality measures differ in terms of the care outcomes they aim to capture?

   _____
   _____
   _____

3. What are some limitations of the current CMS quality measurement system, and how might these impact residents and their families?

   _____
   _____
   _____

4. In what ways does the Resident Assessment Instrument/Minimum Data Set (RAI/MDS) support the goals of quality improvement in nursing homes?

5. How can the insights gained from site visits complement data from tools like Medicare.gov's Care Compare when evaluating nursing homes for a loved one?

NEXTGEN NCLEX STYLE QUESTIONS

1. How does the CMS use quality measures in nursing homes? (Select all that apply)
    a. To provide evidence of abuse in nursing homes
    b. To provide transparency and accountability on nursing home performance
    c. To support facilities in identifying areas for improvement
    d. To close down nursing homes with repeated violations in providing quality care

2. Which tool is used by nursing homes to gather data for quality measures related to residents' clinical conditions, functional abilities, and emotional well-being?
    a. Resident Assessment Instrument/Minimum Data Set (RAI/MDS)
    b. Medicare Quality Review System (MQRS)
    c. Resident Health Evaluation Tool (RHET)
    d. National Nursing Home Assessment Guide (NNHAG)

3. What is one purpose of using the quality measure data in nursing homes?
    a. To replace state inspections in nursing homes
    b. To create new regulations for nursing homes
    c. To eliminate low-performing nursing homes from the CMS system
    d. To help interdisciplinary teams prioritize resources and make improvements

4. How are quality measures categorized in nursing homes based on residents' length of stay?

    a. Temporary and permanent measures

    b. Acute and extended care measures

    c. Short- and long-term measures

    d. Inpatient and outpatient measures

5. Which online tool provided by CMS helps consumers compare nursing homes based on quality measures?

    a. Care Compare

    b. Health Quality Finder

    c. Medicare Facility Guide

    d. Nursing Home Locator

CASE STUDY: Choosing a Quality Nursing Home for a Loved One With Dementia

Scenario

Ms. Ann Wong is seeking a nursing home for her 90-year-old mother, Mrs. Linda Chen, who has advanced dementia and recently suffered a fall that limits her mobility. Mrs. Chen needs a facility that can provide safe, supportive care focused on both her physical needs and her quality of life. Ms. Wong wants a nursing home where her mother's risk of rehospitalization is minimized and where the staff supports her mother's independence as much as possible. She begins researching local nursing homes and comes across Sunrise Haven, which has recently made improvements in several quality measures related to short-stay residents.

Action

Ms. Wong learns that Sunrise Haven has been actively working to reduce its rehospitalization rates and to improve functional outcomes for residents through a Performance Improvement Project. She speaks with the nursing home administrator, Sarah, who shares details about the quality improvement efforts the facility has made over the past few months. Ms. Wong is impressed by the following initiatives:

1. **Interdisciplinary communication:** Sarah explains that the staff at Sunrise Haven holds daily meetings where nursing and rehabilitation teams discuss each resident's status and goals. This practice helps ensure that all team members are aware of residents' needs, including functional goals that are often overlooked in dementia care.

2. **Staff training in dementia care and mobility support:** To support residents like Mrs. Chen, who need mobility assistance and person-centered care, Sunrise Haven has implemented ongoing training for staff. Training includes techniques for safe transfers, personalized mobility exercises, and nonpharmacological strategies for managing dementia-related behaviors. This approach reassures Ms. Wong that her mother will be cared for by knowledgeable staff who are committed to Mrs. Chen's safety and well-being.

3. **Family involvement and discharge planning:** Although Mrs. Chen's dementia limits her ability to communicate, Jessica values being part of her care decisions. Sunrise Haven emphasizes family involvement in care planning and has a structured discharge follow-up program to monitor residents' progress and prevent issues that could lead to rehospitalization. Ms. Wong appreciates that the team will keep her informed and include her in decisions about her mother's care.

4. **Quality-of-life enhancements:** Sunrise Haven has adopted quality measures that prioritize residents' mental and emotional well-being, recognizing that quality care for residents with dementia goes beyond physical health. This includes creating a more home-like environment with sensory activities, quiet spaces, and opportunities for social engagement, even for those with limited mobility.

Outcome

Ms. Wong decides to admit Mrs. Chen to Sunrise Haven, confident that the facility's recent focus on quality improvement measures aligns with her mother's needs. Within her first month, Mrs. Chen shows signs of better mood and mobility, and Ms. Wong feels assured knowing that the nursing home's team is dedicated to her mother's safety, comfort, and quality of life.

Questions

Your instructor may use these questions as a group activity and class discussion, so consider the questions, record your responses below, and bring them to class.

For activities that will be done in class, as discussions or group activities, it is still beneficial to do some reflection before class to prepare.

1. Why was interdisciplinary communication important in Ms. Wong's decision to choose Sunrise Haven?

_____

_____

_____

2. How did staff training in dementia care impact Ms. Wong's confidence in Sunrise Haven?

3. Why is family involvement in care planning important, especially for residents with dementia?

4. What quality-of-life improvements were implemented at Sunrise Haven to support residents with dementia?

5. How do the QI efforts at Sunrise Haven demonstrate a commitment to both safety and person-centered care?

IN-CLASS ACTIVITIES OR ASSIGNMENTS

Your instructor may assign these as in-class activities or as reflection activities done outside of class.

For activities that will be done in class, as discussions or group activities, it is still beneficial to do some reflection before class to prepare.

Learning Activity: Research Evaluating Quality Nursing Home Care

This individual research and writing assignment is designed to provide students with a hands-on experience evaluating nursing home quality, a critical skill for supporting informed decision-making in long-term care.

Objectives

- Evaluate the quality of nursing homes using online tools
- Evaluate the quality of nursing homes using site visits
- Make informed decisions about long-term care for older adults

Materials needed: Podcast episode, Nursing Home Quality Checklist, Medicare.gov's Care Compare website (links provided by instructor)

Assignment Instructions

1. Listen to the assigned podcast episode "Nursing Home: How to Choose a GOOD One (and Avoid a BAD One)" at https://www.youtube.com/watch?v=f19-hdrIlK4. This episode covers essential considerations when evaluating nursing home quality, such as safety, staffing, resident care, and family satisfaction. While listening, take notes on the key indicators of a quality nursing home and warning signs of a poorly performing one. These notes will help guide your approach in later parts of this assignment.

2. Next, select three local nursing homes using Medicare.gov's Care Compare website. Ensure that all three facilities provide similar types of care and services (e.g., memory care, rehabilitation) to make a fair comparison.

3. Based on the Care Compare analysis, select one high-performing and one low-performing nursing home from the three. Schedule a visit to each facility, if possible, and bring a copy of the Nursing Home Quality Checklist to complete during each visit.

4. During the visits, use the Nursing Home Quality Checklist to document observations on the facility's environment, interactions with staff and residents, cleanliness, safety measures, and any other relevant factors. Pay close attention to how each facility aligns (or does not align) with the quality measures noted on Care Compare.

5. Write a two-page reflective paper after completing the visits. The paper should discuss:

    - Your experience comparing the two facilities and how the in-person visit either confirmed or challenged your initial impressions from Care Compare

    - The rationale for choosing one nursing home over the other, including how both quantitative data (Care Compare scores) and qualitative factors (observations from your site visits) influenced your decision

    - Any additional insights gained about evaluating nursing home quality and your thoughts on how these evaluations impact resident care and family peace of mind

APPLICATION OF CONTENT IN THE CLINICAL AND/OR SIMULATION SETTING: Using the NASEM Model of Quality in Nursing Homes to Design a QI Program to Reduce Resident Weight Loss

Simulation & Role-Play Activity

In this simulation, students will role-play as an interdisciplinary team tasked with designing a quality improvement (QI) program to reduce resident weight loss in a nursing home. Using NASEM's conceptual model of quality in nursing homes, students will identify root causes of weight loss and develop strategies to improve nutritional outcomes and quality of life for residents.

Objectives

This simulation will help students apply a structured QI framework within a nursing home setting, emphasizing interdisciplinary collaboration, person-centered care, and the practical application of quality measures to improve resident health outcomes.

Materials needed:

- NASEM's Conceptual Model of Quality in Nursing Homes
- Nursing Home Quality Checklist (for reference)
- Mini Nutritional Assessment (MNA) Screening Tool

Description

Scenario: Bright Horizons Nursing Home has experienced a rising rate of unintended weight loss among its long-stay residents, particularly those with dementia and limited mobility. The nursing home administrator has directed the quality improvement team to develop a plan that addresses this issue, aligns with NASEM's conceptual model of quality, and promotes resident-centered care.

Students will role-play as members of an interdisciplinary QI team, including roles such as a nurse, dietitian, social worker, physical therapist, and nursing home administrator. They will identify potential causes of weight loss, propose interventions, and create an implementation plan using NASEM's model, which emphasizes person-centered care, effective communication, empowered staff, and a supportive environment.

Roles:

1. Nurse: Provides insights on daily resident care, monitors resident intake, and assesses skin integrity and weight trends.
2. Dietitian: Evaluates nutritional intake and dietary needs and provides recommendations for meal planning and nutritional interventions.
3. Social worker: Focuses on understanding residents' social and emotional needs, especially those with cognitive impairments.

4. Physical therapist: Assesses resident mobility and collaborates on interventions that encourage physical activity to stimulate appetite.

5. Nursing home administrator: Oversees resources, policies, and staffing and ensures QI initiatives align with regulatory requirements and facility standards.

Role-Play Activity

Your instructor will lead an in-class role-playing activity to explore possible responses to the scenario.

Debriefing Questions

Your instructor may use these questions as a group activity and class discussion, so consider the questions, record your responses below, and bring them to class.

For activities that will be done in class, as discussions or group activities, it is still beneficial to do some reflection before class to prepare.

1. How did NASEM's model help shape your plan and keep the focus on resident-centered care?

_____

_____

_____

_____

2. What challenges did you encounter in designing interventions within a nursing home setting?

_____

_____

_____

_____

3. What did you learn about how each role contributes to a comprehensive QI program and how team collaboration is essential in long-term care?

_____

_____

_____

_____

CHAPTER 13

NURSING HOME HEALTH INFORMATION TECHNOLOGY

–Andrea Sillner, PhD, RN, GCNS-BC; Kiernan Riley, PhD, BSN, RN; Kalei Crimi, PhD, RN

BRIEF CHAPTER SUMMARY

Health information technology (HIT) in the nursing home setting offers several strengths, including improved care coordination, enhanced patient safety through medication tracking and clinical decision support, and better communication among interdisciplinary teams. HIT systems, such as electronic health records (EHRs), help streamline documentation and ensure that all relevant health information is easily accessible, reducing the risk of errors (Centers for Medicare & Medicaid Services, 2020). However, there are limitations, such as the high costs of implementation and maintenance, limited interoperability between different systems, and challenges related to staff training and adoption (American Health Information Management Association, 2020). Additionally, technical issues, such as system downtimes or user resistance, can hinder the effectiveness of HIT in improving care delivery (HealthIT.gov, 2021).

> **CHAPTER LEARNING OUTCOMES**
> - Introduce the nursing student and staff to nursing home HIT
> - Describe the policies affecting the design and utilization of HIT in nursing homes
> - Discuss the advantages of HIT for quality of care and efficiencies in the nursing home

DISCUSSION QUESTIONS

Discussion Topic: Barriers and Facilitators of Health Information Technology in the Nursing Home

Your instructor may use these questions as a group activity and class discussion, so consider the questions, record your responses below, and bring them to class.

Objective

In this discussion, learners will gain a deeper understanding of the barriers and facilitators to effective HIT use in the nursing home setting. Identifying these factors helps to clarify how the nursing home can address obstacles and capitalize on advantages to improve patient care and staff workflows.

General Discussion Question

During your clinical experience in the nursing home, what barriers and facilitators did you observe related to the use of HIT? Reflect on how these factors impacted patient care, communication, and workflow. How can the nursing home address the barriers and leverage the facilitators to enhance the adoption and effectiveness of HIT? Use the space below to record your notes.

_____

_____

_____

_____

Follow-Up Questions to Guide the Discussion

Barriers to HIT Use

1. What challenges did you notice regarding access to or training on HIT systems (e.g., EHRs, medication management systems, etc.)?

   _____

   _____

   _____

2. Did you observe any issues with system interoperability (e.g., difficulties in sharing information between the nursing home and external providers)?

   _____

   _____

   _____

3. Were there any technical difficulties, such as system downtime or slow load times, that hindered the use of HIT?

   _____

   _____

   _____

4. How did staff workload or staffing levels impact the effective use of HIT? Did the workload create challenges in utilizing HIT systems efficiently?

_____

_____

_____

_____

5. Were there any concerns regarding data privacy or security that affected the use of HIT (e.g., reluctance to input sensitive information into the system)?

_____

_____

_____

Facilitators of HIT Use

6. What features of HIT systems helped improve communication between staff, residents, and external providers?

_____

_____

_____

7. Were there any tools or systems in place that supported interdisciplinary collaboration (e.g., shared calendars, messaging features, alert systems)?

_____

_____

_____

8. Did you observe any examples of HIT being used to enhance patient safety (e.g., medication alerts, clinical decision support)?

9. How did leadership or organizational support contribute to the effective use of HIT (e.g., providing adequate training, ensuring resources are available)?

10. Were there any positive outcomes or efficiencies observed as a result of HIT implementation (e.g., quicker documentation, fewer errors, better care coordination)?

Improving HIT Use in the Nursing Home

11. Based on your observations, how can the nursing home address the barriers to HIT use? What practical steps can be taken to improve staff engagement, training, and system reliability?

12. How can the nursing home further leverage the facilitators to optimize HIT systems and improve resident care?

13. What role do you think staff involvement and feedback play in enhancing the effectiveness of HIT? How can nursing home leadership encourage a culture of continuous improvement with HIT?

NEXTGEN NCLEX STYLE QUESTIONS

1. A nurse in a nursing home is using the EHR system to update a resident's care plan. The nurse receives a notification from the system alerting them that the attending physician has ordered a new medication for the resident. The nurse is unsure of the medication's dosage and administration schedule. Which of the following actions should the nurse take to ensure safe and effective communication with the interdisciplinary care team?

    a. Contact the pharmacy department directly through the EHR messaging system for clarification.

    b. Send a secure message to the attending physician through the EHR system asking for clarification on the medication order.

    c. Administer the medication as ordered by the physician, assuming the dosage is correct.

    d. Wait until the physician makes a physical visit to clarify the medication order.

2. A nursing home nurse is using a health information exchange (HIE) system to share a resident's health data with a hospital team for an upcoming procedure. The resident has a complex medical history, including chronic diseases and recent surgeries. Which of the following should the nurse prioritize when sending the resident's data through the HIE to ensure the hospital team receives the most relevant and accurate information?

    a. Include all of the resident's historical medical data, even if it is not directly related to the upcoming procedure.

    b. Send a hard copy of the resident's chart to the hospital along with the electronic data for reference.

    c. Allow the hospital team to access the full EHR and make their own decisions about what information is necessary.

    d. Ensure the data is up to date, clearly organized, and includes only information pertinent to the upcoming procedure.

3. A nursing home nurse receives an alert via the health information system that a resident's lab results indicate an elevated potassium level. The system advises notifying the attending physician immediately. Which action should the nurse take to ensure the proper use of the HIT system to communicate this critical finding?

    a. Use the system's secure messaging feature to notify the attending physician of the elevated potassium level and request further orders.

    b. Immediately document the lab results in the resident's chart and wait for the physician's next scheduled visit.

    c. Call the physician's office directly and leave a voicemail message regarding the lab results.

    d. Post the lab result on the nurse's station bulletin board for all staff to see and address it during the next care team meeting.

4. A nurse in a nursing home is coordinating care for a resident with a wound care specialist, physical therapist, and dietician. The nurse plans to update the interdisciplinary team about the resident's progress using the facility's HIT system. Which of the following actions should the nurse take to ensure effective communication across the care team?

    a. Leave detailed notes in the resident's chart but do not directly communicate with the team members through the HIT system.

    b. Use the EHR system's team communication feature to send an update that includes the resident's current condition, treatment plan, and any relevant concerns to each team member.

    c. Only communicate with the wound care specialist through the EHR system, as they are the primary care provider.

    d. Wait until the next interdisciplinary team meeting to provide updates and discuss the resident's care.

5. A nurse at a nursing home is updating a resident's EHR when they notice that another healthcare professional has accessed the resident's record without permission. The nurse is concerned about potential violations of data privacy. What is the nurse's best course of action in this situation?

   a. Ignore the incident, as it is unlikely to have been intentional, and continue with the care process.

   b. Confront the healthcare professional directly and ask why they accessed the record.

   c. Report the unauthorized access immediately to the facility's HIPAA compliance officer and document the incident in the appropriate system.

   d. Delete the resident's health information from the system to prevent further access.

OpenAI (2024) was used in the formatting of NCLEX style questions based on Alexander (2023).

CASE STUDY: Coordinating a Specialist Appointment Using Health Information Technology in the Nursing Home

Patient Profile

Name: Mrs. Eleanor Thompson

Age: 82

Admission date: Six months ago

Reason for admission: Mrs. Thompson was admitted to the nursing home after suffering a stroke, which led to significant mobility impairment and mild cognitive decline. She also has a history of hypertension, diabetes, and osteoarthritis.

Chronic conditions:
- Hypertension (managed with medication)
- Type 2 diabetes (requires insulin)
- Osteoarthritis (affecting both knees)
- Mild cognitive impairment (unable to fully manage medications independently)

Current medications:
- Lisinopril 10 mg daily
- Metformin 500 mg twice a day
- Insulin sliding scale for blood sugar management
- Acetaminophen as needed for pain relief

Functional status: Mrs. Thompson is dependent on staff for mobility and requires assistance with most activities of daily living. She is able to engage in conversations but has difficulty remembering appointments or instructions.

Scenario

Mrs. Thompson needs to see a rheumatologist for an evaluation of her osteoarthritis, which has been worsening. The appointment is scheduled for 30 days from today. She requires transportation to and from the specialist's office, and the nursing home staff must ensure all aspects of this appointment are communicated and coordinated effectively using HIT.

The nurse assigned to Mrs. Thompson, Nurse Johnson, needs to ensure a smooth transition of care for her upcoming rheumatology appointment in 30 days. Nurse Johnson uses the EHR system and interdepartmental communication forms to coordinate with various team members and external entities involved in the appointment.

Action

1. Nurse Johnson completes the interdepartmental communication form:

    Action: Nurse Johnson logs into the EHR system and fills out an interdepartmental communication form to inform the social worker, transportation coordinator, and other relevant team members about the upcoming appointment. The form includes details such as the appointment date, time, purpose of the visit, and any special needs for Mrs. Thompson.

    Information shared:

    a. Mrs. Thompson's personal details (name, room number)

    b. Appointment details (specialist, appointment time, transportation needs)

    c. Relevant health information (medications, mobility needs)

    d. Contact information for the family member (daughter) who will be available on the day of the appointment

2. Communication with the social worker:

    Action: The social worker receives the form via the EHR messaging system and reviews Mrs. Thompson's need for transportation to the specialist's office. The social worker is tasked with coordinating the transportation for the appointment. They contact the family and the transportation company to confirm the arrangements.

    HIT use: The social worker uses the EHR messaging system to communicate with Nurse Johnson and update the team on the confirmed transportation schedule. The transportation service is scheduled via the nursing home's internal calendar system, which automatically updates all relevant staff.

3. Scheduling the appointment with the specialist's office:

   Action: Nurse Johnson calls the rheumatology specialist's office to schedule the appointment. The nurse verifies the date and time and confirms that the appointment will require transportation. Nurse Johnson then enters the appointment details into the nursing home's EHR system.

   HIT use: The EHR system is updated with the appointment details and linked to Mrs. Thompson's medical record. The specialist's office sends an electronic confirmation of the appointment back to the nursing home, which is added to the organizational calendar.

4. Coordination with the nursing home's calendar:

   Action: The appointment details are added to the nursing home's shared calendar, ensuring all relevant nursing and interdisciplinary staff are aware of Mrs. Thompson's absence on the day of the appointment. This includes updating the nursing shifts, ensuring staff availability for medication administration, and making any adjustments to care plans as necessary.

   HIT use: The calendar system allows for easy access by all staff to review upcoming appointments and adjust care assignments. Notifications are sent to relevant parties (nursing, social work, etc.).

5. Communication with the resident and family:

   Action: The social worker contacts Mrs. Thompson's daughter (family contact) using the EHR's secure messaging system to inform her about the specialist appointment and confirm any additional needs or questions. Nurse Johnson also discusses the appointment with Mrs. Thompson to ensure she understands the visit and what will happen.

   HIT use: The secure messaging system ensures that the family can be kept up to date with all details, reducing the likelihood of confusion on the day of the appointment. Mrs. Thompson's daughter confirms she will accompany her mother to the appointment.

Questions

Your instructor may use these questions as a group activity and class discussion, so consider the questions, record your responses below, and bring them to class.

For activities that will be done in class, as discussions or group activities, it is still beneficial to do some reflection before class to prepare.

1. Barriers to effective use of HIT: What are the potential barriers to effective use of HIT in the scenario above?

   _____
   _____
   _____

2. Improving care transitions using HIT: How can the nursing home improve the process of care transitions and communication across teams using HIT?

   _____
   _____
   _____

3. Addressing technology and workflow gaps: What gaps in technology or workflow could disrupt the coordination of the appointment for Mrs. Thompson, and how can these gaps be addressed?

   _____
   _____
   _____

4. Role of the nurse in coordinating care transitions: What role does Nurse Johnson play in ensuring that HIT systems are used effectively during this care transition?

   _____
   _____
   _____

Conclusion

In this case study, the use of HIT helps to coordinate care for Mrs. Thompson, facilitating communication among the interdisciplinary team, external specialists, and her family. However, barriers to effective use of HIT—such as interoperability issues, access to technology, and workforce readiness—can hinder smooth transitions. Identifying and addressing these barriers is crucial for improving the quality of care during transitions and ensuring that all parties involved are informed and prepared for the appointment. By refining workflows and enhancing technology infrastructure, nursing homes can improve care transitions and ensure better outcomes for their residents.

IN-CLASS ACTIVITIES OR ASSIGNMENTS

Your instructor may assign these as in-class activities or as reflection activities done outside of class.

For activities that will be done in class, as discussions or group activities, it is still beneficial to do some reflection before class to prepare.

Learning Activity: Identifying and Defining Common Health Information Technology Terms in the Nursing Home Setting

This assignment may be assigned as a written assignment, an in-class assignment, or a short quiz.

Assignment Instructions

HIT plays a vital role in improving the quality, safety, and efficiency of care in the nursing home setting. As a nursing professional, understanding the terminology related to HIT is essential to effectively navigate HIT systems and improve communication, care coordination, and patient safety.

In this assignment, you will identify and define common terms related to HIT used in the nursing home. This will help you become familiar with key concepts and the language of HIT systems, which are integral to your practice.

1. Research: Using textbooks, scholarly articles, or reputable online sources (such as government health websites or nursing journals), identify and define 10–15 common HIT terms used in the nursing home setting. For each term, provide a brief (one-to-two sentence) definition.

2. References: Include three to five scholarly references that you used to define these terms. Ensure that you use APA format for citations and references.

3. Submission: Submit your completed assignment to the course's online platform or email as your instructor indicates.

Example Answer Entry

Clinical decision support

Definition: Tools embedded in HIT systems that provide alerts, reminders, or recommendations to assist healthcare providers in making evidence-based clinical decisions

Source: Institute of Medicine, 2013

Learning Activity: Points of Failure in Health Information Technology in the Nursing Home Setting

This may be assigned as a written assignment or reflection in an in-person or online course or in a discussion board type of activity. The questions can be addressed together or independently.

Assignment Instructions

HIT plays a critical role in improving the quality of care, communication, and safety in the nursing home setting. However, various challenges exist in effectively implementing and sustaining HIT systems in these environments. In this assignment, you will explore the barriers identified by Alexander and Mullen (2023) that prevent successful integration of HIT in nursing homes and how these issues affect interdisciplinary care and patient outcomes.

Step 1: Read the article by Alexander and Mullen (2023) that outlines the following four points of failure for HIT in the nursing home setting:

1. Conflicting policy and reforms that do not benefit all sections of healthcare
2. Lack of infrastructure to implement and sustain HIT in nursing homes
3. Growing time between creation of HIT systems and implementation of data sharing
4. Lack of workforce readiness to adopt HIT in nursing homes

Step 2: After reviewing the article and reflecting on the content, write a detailed report that addresses the following questions:

1. Identify and explain how conflicting policies at the federal or state level can hinder the effective use of HIT in nursing homes. Discuss examples of policy reforms that may benefit hospitals or outpatient care but do not address the unique needs of nursing homes.

    Points to address:

    a. How do policies favoring acute care settings over long-term care settings affect HIT implementation in nursing homes?

    b. What are some examples of current policies that may negatively impact the ability of nursing homes to adopt HIT effectively?

2. Describe the challenges nursing homes face in developing and maintaining the infrastructure necessary to support HIT systems. This can include technological, financial, and organizational barriers.

    Points to address:

    a. What are some of the key infrastructure barriers (e.g., outdated technology, lack of internet connectivity) in nursing homes that hinder the implementation of HIT?

b. Discuss the financial strain nursing homes may experience when trying to implement and sustain HIT systems.

  c. How does the physical layout of many nursing homes impact the implementation of HIT systems?

3. Discuss the delay between the creation of new HIT systems and their actual implementation in nursing homes. Why does this lag time occur, and what are the consequences for patient care and communication among the interdisciplinary team?

   Points to address:

   a. What are some examples of HIT systems that are not being implemented in a timely manner within nursing homes?

   b. How does this delay impact the quality of care and communication between nursing home staff and other healthcare providers?

   c. What can be done to accelerate the adoption and integration of HIT systems in nursing homes?

4. Evaluate the readiness of the nursing home workforce to adopt and utilize HIT systems. What are the training and support gaps that prevent staff from fully utilizing technology in patient care and communication?

   Points to address:

   a. What are some barriers that nursing home staff face in terms of adopting and using HIT (e.g., lack of training, resistance to change, unfamiliarity with technology)?

   b. How can nursing homes improve staff readiness to use HIT systems effectively? Discuss strategies for providing ongoing training and support.

   c. What role do leadership and management play in preparing the workforce to embrace HIT?

5. In your conclusion, summarize the main points of failure identified in your report. Reflect on potential solutions or strategies that could help address these challenges and improve the adoption and use of HIT in nursing homes. Consider how resolving these issues could improve patient care, communication among care teams, and overall outcomes for residents.

APPLICATION OF CONTENT IN THE CLINICAL AND/OR SIMULATION SETTING: Post-Clinical Reflection on Health Information Technology Usage

Your instructor may assign this as a debriefing discussion in an in-person or online course or as a written assignment.

Debriefing Questions

Your instructor will ask you to reflect on your clinical experience and identify and describe all the ways HIT was utilized during your time in the nursing home setting.

Your instructor may use the following questions as a group activity and class discussion, so consider the questions, record your responses below, and bring them to class.

For activities that will be done in class, as discussions or group activities, it is still beneficial to do some reflection before class to prepare.

1. Did you observe the use of EHRs for documenting patient care or sharing information with interdisciplinary team members? What did you observe?

2. Were any HIT tools used for scheduling appointments, managing medication administration, or tracking patient outcomes? Which tools were used?

3. How did technology support communication with external providers, such as specialists or pharmacies?

4. Were there any instances where HIT was used to support patient safety (e.g., medication alerts, clinical decision support)? If so, describe the instances.

_____

_____

_____

_____

5. Did you encounter any challenges or barriers to effective use of HIT (e.g., system access issues, lack of training, technology malfunctions)? If so, describe the challenges or barriers you encountered.

_____

_____

_____

_____

6. What suggestions do you have for improving the integration and use of HIT in the nursing home setting?

_____

_____

_____

_____

REFERENCES

Alexander, G. L. (2023). Nursing home health information technology. In J. Reifsnyder, A. Kolanowski, & J. Dunbar-Jacob (Eds.), *Practice & leadership in nursing homes: Building on academic-practice partnerships* (pp. 355–372). Sigma Theta Tau International.

Alexander, G. L., & McMullen, T. (2023). Probing into federal policies and National Academies' recommendations to adopt health information technology in all U.S. nursing homes. *Public Policy & Aging Report, 33*(Suppl_1), S28–S34. https://doi.org/10.1093/ppar/prac026

American Health Information Management Association. (2020). *The benefits and challenges of health information technology in nursing homes.* https://www.ahima.org

Assistant Secretary for Technology Policy. (2021). *Health information technology basics.* https://www.healthit.gov/topic/health-it-basics

Centers for Medicare & Medicaid Services. (2020). *Meaningful use of electronic health records.* https://www.cms.gov/Regulations-and-Guidance/Legislation/EHRIncentivePrograms

OpenAI. (2024). *ChatGPT* (December version) [Large language model]. https://chat.openai.com/